Table of Contents

Dedication	5
Introduction	7
Chapter 1: California Dreaming	9
Chapter 2: The Early Years	17
Chapter 3: Irreconcilable Differences	23
Chapter 4: What Was I Thinking?	27
Chapter 5: On the Move	33
Chapter 6: Charting a New Course	41
Chapter 7: True Friends Last a Lifetime	47
Chapter 8: True Friends Last a Lifetime, Part 2	57
Chapter 9: Life Takes Its Course	69
Chapter 10: Tumultuous Years	75
Chapter 11: Baby, It's Cold Outside	87
Chapter 12: Big Changes	91
Chapter 13: Saying Goodbye	97
Chapter 14: Alone Again	101
Chapter 15: Spring Fling	107
Chapter 16: Escape Hatch	113
Chapter 17: Derailed	121
Chapter 18: Bombshell	129
Chapter 19: Midnight Confession	137
Chapter 20: Gone	145
Chapter 21: Sleepless in Louisiana	153
Chapter 22: One Day at a Time	159
Chapter 23: Come October	165
Epilogue	175

For Jeremy
(1975-2018)
You are the bright star
in my universe.

Introduction

This is going to be the hardest thing I've ever done. Keep in mind, I say this after having lost everything in Hurricane Katrina in 2005—including my husband's and my jobs, and then, eighteen months later, losing my wonderful, loving husband.

Then came the unbelievably painful reality, that my son—my only child, my best friend, my roommate, my business partner—was gone. Jeremy was dead at forty-three.

As I write this, I think about a lady who heard my story in a public setting and as she left, handed me a folded piece of paper and smiled. When I got outside, I opened the paper and read her handwritten note, "My strategy for getting through hardships–realizing that I will never have to go through anything this hard ever again."

I took a deep breath and realized that I'd gone through the worst thing a mother can ever face; the death of her only child. And yet I'm still "alive."

I say "alive" in quotes because most of the time, I'm not living. Instead, I'm standing in the void of eternity, wondering how long I have to wait to be reunited with my precious son again.

I've certainly thought about the alternatives: not taking my maintenance medications or just swallowing the entire bottle of anxiety meds, which is the only thing that brings me sleep because when I close my eyes, the memory of Jeremy's death replays in head over and over again like an old record skipping on a scratch.

I don't know if it's lack of courage or tenacity that tells me this is not the way to go. I have a deep-seated need to share my story in hopes of saving other parents this grief. Unfortunately, I know there are a lot of us out there. But if I can prevent just one person from experiencing the inexplicable pain I'm going through, if I can prevent one child from disappearing down the path that consumed my Jeremy, it will bring me some sort of peace.

So, here's my story. But for the grace of God, it could be anyone's…

1

California Dreaming

It was the summer of 1971.

Kansas just didn't cut it for me and my friend Gail anymore. Just like Dorothy dreamed of a more exciting life in *The Wizard of Oz*, Gail and I did too. But our "Oz" was the storybook setting we thought existed on the West Coast. California. The decision of two adventurous, barely twenty-two-year-olds, with the life experience of a goldfish, led to the events that shaped the rest of my life.

Dreaming of blue skies, sandy beaches, movie stars and all the magic found in a tourist ad for California, our decision was made. When Gail and I concocted our inspirational plan, all we had was $150 between us and a 1967 Opel Kadett that used more oil than gasoline. We hadn't bothered to sort out the minor details of how we were going to travel 1,620 miles. Not to mention find a place to stay once we reached Dreamland. Our lack of resources never entered our star-struck minds.

Sleeping in the car, surviving on bologna and white bread sandwiches, Gail and I eventually arrived in Los Angeles with $6.75 left from our travel budget. Normally, that's the makings of a dangerous situation that could end very badly. Think about it: no place to sleep, no money to buy food, no jobs. This situation was far from the plot of a successful, happy-ending "Lifetime" movie. Instead, it had the makings of a "true crime" documentary.

Fortunately for us, Gail's ex-husband from a short-lived marriage lived in the LA area. After some detective work and spending a chunk of our $6.75 in pay phones, we were lucky enough to find a contact number for Bob. And Bob was kind enough to take us in until we could find jobs and support ourselves. Although he never said a thing, I knew Bob was hoping that this was a chance to rekindle his relationship with Gail. But whatever the reason for his generosity, we were grateful for it.

Not long after our arrival, both Gail and I were able to find work that allowed us to pay our way. Mine was in a neighborhood beer joint. It was the kind of place that seemed lost in time with its round, red vinyl covered seats at a long bar, a juke box on the back wall near the rear exit and a pool table in the middle of the room. The place was so small that it was packed when twenty people showed up on Friday and Saturday night!

It didn't take long for the regulars to spread the word that the grandmotherly woman who'd tended bar for years retired and had been replaced by a cute, twenty-two-year-old wearing hot pants and go-go boots. In 1967, they were the height of fashion and I was a fashion plate.

Most of the patrons were much older than me (read that as "old men"), so when a young guy came into the bar on a boisterous Friday night, he got my attention. On one such evening, this particular man ordered a draft beer, which I delivered with a smile. He was good looking but very quiet. He didn't seem to interact with anyone, maybe because the crowd was so much older.

I decided that there was no reason to just watch this handsome stranger and wait for him to get up the nerve to strike up a conversation with me. After all, chatting up the customers was part of my job. Hair down to his shoulders and a shy look on his face, he piqued my curiosity. That's how and when I met David.

•

Months later, when Gail decided to return to Kansas to the boyfriend she'd left behind, I chose to stay and live with David. About six months later, we got married. David and I had a small wedding in a chapel with family and a modest reception at his brother's home.

I was happy but homesick. Several months later, I talked David into moving to Kansas City where my family and friends were. The promise of an immediate job sealed the deal for him. In LA, we sold what we had, including David's 1965 Triumph motorcycle, his pride and joy. We bought a used car, packed up and headed east.

At first, David and I rented an apartment in the neighborhood where I grew up. But before long, we heard that the elderly lady who lived in a lovely two-story house her husband had built in the 1940s was leaving her home. The place was perfect. Just around the corner from the home where I grew up, the yard connected with my parent's backyard by way of a gate. The house cost $7,000 and the lady carried the mortgage note herself at a very low interest rate.

It sounded perfect. The woman wanted to sell to a young couple who would raise their family there, much like she and her husband had. David and I fit the bill. We moved in with our scanty belongings and gathered used and hand-me-down furniture to begin making a home. Since we were both working, it wasn't long before David and I could start replacing the odds and ends with new furniture. It was a big benefit to us that Mom lived just beyond the backyard gate. She cooked a great supper every night and always had plenty for anyone who stopped by. You can be sure that David and I "stopped by" often.

Our weekends were spent with my lifelong friends: girls I went all through school with, and their husbands. We became what we called "the Tribe." Everyone gathered at one of our homes and we cooked and talked and laughed together, late into the night.

•

As the Tribe grew, our late nights became fewer and fewer. Two couples delivered healthy baby boys over the next two years. One couple already had a little girl, Robin. And in May of 1974, I found out that our baby would be the fourth child of the Tribe.

Pregnancy was a breeze for me. The only thing I couldn't stomach was Chinese food; I couldn't make it past the smell. This was annoying at best since Chinese food was one of my favorites—and it's ironic that it turned out to be a favorite of my son Jeremy's as well.

In 1974, expectant parents didn't find out the sex of their child until they were actually born. Routine ultra sounds weren't a thing back then. And honestly, I think not knowing was more exciting than knowing.

January 18, 1975 was the best day of my life!

At 5:40 a.m. on a bright winter Saturday, Jeremy Joseph made his debut. In the mid-Seventies, hospitals treated mothers delivering babies more like patients. Moms and dads-to-be waited out the time in a "labor room" until the nurses determined that you were ready to be moved to a delivery room.

During this first stage of labor, it was common for pain medication to be given to the expectant mom, whether she wanted it or not. Being wheeled into what looked like an operating room did not make me feel relaxed, so this nervous, first-time mom took whatever meds she was offered, no questions asked. Due to the drugs, my memory is foggy as to everything that went on during Jeremy's delivery. At some point, they put a mask over my nose and mouth and I slipped in and out of awareness.

When they brought my son to me for the first time, I immediately noticed that he had a bright, red mark on the top of his head. Concerned, I asked about it. The nurse explained that Jeremy had become "hung up" by my pelvic bone and the doctor had to use forceps to deliver him. So, that was the reason for the red mark! I breathed a sigh of relief.

What I remember most just after Jeremy's birth is a nurse coming into the recovery room and telling David and I that they were waiting for a bigger room to become available so they could move me into it. Why did I need such a big room? It seemed that the Tribe had descended upon the waiting room after being notified of the impending birth of a new family member. As was our group's custom, they all went to the hospital, no matter what time it was.

Spending three days in the hospital was the required stay at that time. Whenever the nurses brought Jeremy to me, I always knew it was the right baby because he had that distinct X on his head from the forceps. I would joke with the nurse and tell her, "Mine's the one with the X!" So, there was no possibility of getting Jeremy mixed up in the nursery. X marks the spot!

•

It was so much fun to bring my beautiful baby boy home to all of our family and friends! People stopped by all day long to meet Jeremy. My dad fell instantly in love with his new grandson. Now, my father was not one to show affection. As a kid, I don't ever remember him hugging us or saying "I love you." My siblings and I knew he loved us but he just didn't know how to show it. My mother, on the other hand, was very jovial and loving.

Dad also didn't like to go out. If mom mentioned that she wanted to visit someone, he generally didn't go along. His likely response was, "They know where we live if they want to see us." So, on the evening of Jeremy's first day at home, the fact that I opened the front door to see my dad smiling broadly, saying "Well, let me see the little rascal!" spoke volumes. It was my dad's way of showing his affection and he grew to love my son dearly. We all did.

One of the most pivotal moments of my life happened when Jeremy was a newborn. I remember holding him close, rocking him in a rocking chair. My son was wrapped tightly in a blanket, happy, content. We were alone. I studied Jeremy's dark eyes and chubby cheeks. He even had my dimple! Right then and there, I made a vow to my son that he would always be the single most important person in my life.

I didn't realize at the time that I'd already made the decision Jeremy would be an only child. I wanted so much for him. I'd seen my sister raising five children and my brothers, three. Yes, it was nice that their kids had siblings but I knew Jeremy would have close childhood playmates with our friends' children. I wanted to be in a position to give Jeremy every opportunity that his dad and I never had. I wanted to spoil him but not spoil him rotten!

2

The Early Years

Other than the usual sleep deprivation every parent experiences with a newborn who wakes up every few hours hungry, Jeremy was an easy child. No colic, no colds or sniffles, not even teething pain! We simply noticed a new tooth had sprouted, no drama or tears.

Maybe Jeremy's pleasant disposition was because I created a large playroom with shelves full of toys to keep him busy. Or maybe it was because he had so much time with extended family lavishing attention on him. But Jeremy was a sweet, loving, easygoing toddler. He shared his toys, never threw a tantrum in a store or otherwise.

Now, I'm not going to say he was an angel—Jeremy spent his fair share of time standing in a corner, the "time out" of the day. But he never gave us any real trouble as a little one.

I like to think this was the start of the gentle, warm, big-hearted man Jeremy grew into. As a child, he was quick to learn and master new tasks. I could tell when he was fairly young that Jeremy was pretty bright. I often told him, "You're going to grow up and be a fabulous lawyer." When people asked why I wanted Jeremy to be a lawyer, I'd respond, "I don't necessarily want him to be a lawyer but if I keep telling him that, I think he'll grow up to be something great."

Sadly, I don't have many special memories of Jeremy with his dad David. There wasn't the strong father/son bond I expected. David didn't seem particularly focused or interested in what Jeremy was up to. This is not to say that David didn't love him because I know he did. But David was never quite the loving father I expected him to be. Maybe this stemmed from the fact that David's father wasn't "present" in his life. Because of David's emotional distance from our son, I'm so grateful for my parents' closeness to Jeremy as well as the Tribe's.

•

Two very important memories of Jeremy as a child stand out in my mind. He must have been about four and five years old. Both memories include his grandfather, my dad.

Now, Grandpa seldom drove. Unbelievably, my mother took him to and from work every day. His interest in driving was only sparked by his desire to entertain Jeremy. Dad worked at a grain elevator, which, on evenings and weekends, was deserted.

At least once a week, Dad loaded Jeremy into the car and the two of them went to explore the grain elevator. Because there were railroad tracks adjacent to the elevator (they were used to ship boxcars full of grain), walking along those rails as dad and Jeremy "hunted" for big game was an exciting adventure.

Grandpa pointed out what surely must be bear tracks. Of course, there were lion and tiger tracks too. Oh my! Jeremy came home from these expeditions wide eyed and excited, telling me how Grandpa had spotted animal tracks. My little guy believed this with all his heart.

When Jeremy got a little older and figured out that maybe they weren't big game tracks after all, it was time for Grandpa to shift gears and introduce him to his favorite hobby; fishing. Friends of the family had a farm about an hour north of the city. There were several acres and lots of ponds filled with all types of fish. Since only family and close friends were permitted to fish there, the fish were plentiful. It was more like fishing in a bath tub. As the saying goes, "It wasn't fishing; it was catching." You were pretty much guaranteed to catch something.

The first time Grandpa took five-year-old Jeremy fishing, he rigged up a rod and reel. This wasn't a kiddie setup, but real, grown-up equipment with a worm and bobber. Grandpa patiently explained that when the bobber went under the water, you had to pull back on the rod to hook the fish. Now that Jeremy was ready, Grandpa could get started bass fishing himself. He preferred using a lure.

There's a difference between bait fishing and lure fishing. The way bass and most other game fish are caught, the lure fishing requires the fisherman to cast out the line and slowly reel it in. This makes the lure to look like a moving, live fish. AKA, supper.

Well, Jeremy must have liked this more active fishing technique because, as my dad told it, Jeremy started reeling in his line and trying to cast it out again and again. I guess he was trying to copy what his granddad was doing.

Grandpa watched Jeremy's method for a bit and finally went to his tackle box. He nosed around in the giant, fold-out silver case that was filled with dozens of lures and supplies. Grandpa grabbed a lure, called Jeremy over and said, "If you're not going to leave your bait in the water, you might as well be fishing with a lure so you can keep reeling it in and practice casting it." Little Jeremy agreed.

That day, that statement, started Jeremy on his lifelong love of fishing. He and Grandpa spent many Sunday afternoons with newspapers spread on the living room carpet going through and cleaning out that big, silver tackle box. Of course, the most impressive lures were fodder for "big fish" stories. The wider Jeremy's eyes grew, the bigger Grandpa's fish story got. It was so wonderful to see my dad and son bonding through fishing.

Jeremy continued to fish throughout his life. His last few trips were with good friends in the Gulf of Mexico just off southern Louisiana. He proudly brought home beautiful red fish to grill. Grilling and smoking fish and meat was Jeremy's only real adventures with cooking, but he was very skilled at both.

•

Sometime between four and five years old, Jeremy began spending lots of time playing in the backyard. Mysteriously, spoons started disappearing from my silverware drawer. When I discovered Jeremy digging holes in the yard with cutlery, I asked, "Why are you digging all these holes in the yard?"

My five-year-old's reply would foretell his future career. "I love the dirt," Jeremy said. "It 'transalizes' me!"

So, it looked like I was going to have an excavator for a son, not a lawyer. And that was fine with me. Just so long as he found a job that transalized him.

For a couple of years after that, every birthday and Christmas, Jeremy's presents included Tonka trucks and heavy play equipment like bulldozers, diggers and dump trucks. When Jeremy tired of playing in the dirt, his Legos and his Star Wars collection, rivaled by none, were his indoor go-to toys. That child loved tinkering. With anything.

T-ball and baseball were the step-up from little boy games. Jeremy was growing into a young man. A couple of the dads decided to organize a ball team. Since we lived in a neighborhood called Northeast (the same one my friends and I grew up in), the team became the Northeast Yankees. Those kids were so stinking cute in their miniature Yankee uniforms! The kids looked like they knew what they were doing but in reality, had no clue. The players were captivated by butterflies, trees, and every other distraction, everything except the ball.

Fortunately, the coaches were all about the kids having a good time so there was none of the scolding or humiliation you often see at young children's sporting events today. The focus was on fun. By some miracle, the Northeast Yankees actually managed to win a game or two!

These were sweet, uncomplicated times. Little did I know how drastically my life would change when Jeremy got older.

3

Irreconcilable Differences

By the time Jeremy was seven, David's and my marriage was not a good one, at least not for me. Because we didn't share the same interests, it was easy to grow in different directions. I'm an extrovert and David's an introvert, and after a while, opposites didn't attract.

Back when Jeremy was four, I took a job as Vice President of Sales for a midsize corporation. David was working as a driver for a distribution company that delivered to fast-food restaurants. My typical work schedule consisted of ten-hour days, five days a week, and the days were very long and stressful. David's job as a trucker allowed for drivers to bid on their runs. As I got busier, David began to cut back on his "bid run" from five days a week to four and eventually, three.

At thirty years old, I felt it was time to make our future. David and I were in a good position to advance our careers, set goals and earn the means to obtain them. But my husband didn't seem to agree. I probably wouldn't have been so critical if David had used his at home time to parent Jeremy. But that's not what happened.

Most days David was home, he sent Jeremy next door to my parents' house so he could "nap." David couldn't seem to complete simple household chores like cleaning up the kitchen after he ate. It was clear he felt it was MY job to look after him; he couldn't even manage to clean up after himself, let alone Jeremy. The few days we spent together, David was withdrawn. He watched TV and barely spoke. If I asked him what was wrong, David's answer was always the same, "Nothing."

However, I did manage to talk David into what I saw as an opportunity for us. Our home was paid for and a house nearby that my brother used to own had become available for purchase. The owner was bent on selling it, and quick, so the deal was a good one. David and I bought the house, got a mortgage and decided to update the place before moving in. Our intention was to rent or sell our first home. Simple enough.

David and I agreed that he could handle the small renovations—like adding tile to the bathroom—in his time off. But he only managed to get it half done. I'm the first to admit that I am NOT a patient person. Once a decision is made, I'm ready to get whatever it is done. I complete the task as soon as I can. But not David.

This impatience translates into me always being on time. Me being thirty minutes late for an appointment would warrant a call to Missing

Persons. David, on the other hand, was always late to everything and put off tasks as long as possible. It was starting to wear thin.

The bottom line is I was totally bored with David. I wasn't in love with him the way I wanted to be in love. And I was exhausted from trying to make things happen by myself. I wondered how long I would last in this unfulfilling marriage.

•

I'm glad to report that Jeremy and his dad had a decent relationship throughout his life. I'm especially happy that during the last few years before David died in 2015, he and Jeremy had several adventures together. Their mutual interest in gold mining led them to take trips to Colorado, Arizona, and other locations out west to spend valuable one-on-one time doing something they both loved.

But unfortunately, Jeremy inherited his father's procrastination gene. Throughout his entire life, our biggest problem was my pushing Jeremy to "Don't put off 'til tomorrow what you can do today." It seldom worked.

Jeremy always got everything done. Eventually. But he was always pushing a deadline to the limit. It actually surprised me that after twenty years of making and adhering to building schedules for multi-million-dollar projects, Jeremy still had difficulty managing his personal time. We lived in our last home together for two-and-a-half years and there were still five or six unpacked boxes in his sitting room when he died.

•

My discontent with David grew to the point that I couldn't take it any longer. I deserved to be happy, didn't I? I deserved to feel fulfilled. I deserved a soul partner, right?

When I told David I wanted a divorce, his reaction wasn't much different than if I had said, "We're having meatloaf for supper." I don't even remember having a discussion about why I wanted to end our marriage. Didn't he care? Wasn't he the least bit curious? I guess not.

My gut feeling was that David was okay with it. Maybe he'd sensed my unhappiness but he gave no indication. There wasn't any pushback from him.

Because I was the one who decided to end our union, I was the one who left. I took Jeremy from the house behind my parents' place and moved to the house we hadn't finished renovating, the house that carried a mortgage. I also took the car we were in the process of paying off and gave David the vehicle that was paid in full. I didn't want to be unfair to him and I certainly didn't want a battle to play out in front of Jeremy.

So, in September 1982, when Jeremy was seven, ten years after marrying, David and I divorced.

4

What Was I Thinking?

Leaving a marriage after ten years, basically due to terminal boredom, I made the awful mistake of boarding the first train to Funville. From summer of 1983 until 1995, many of the things I did, I wouldn't do again in a million years. In fact, I find it difficult to reconcile that I did them at all. I thought I was a strong, independent woman with a good career, and at the very least, common sense. But somehow, I lost myself to my own vulnerabilities and fears.

•

Jeremy and I moved to our new address easily enough without a difficult transition. The following spring, my nieces Shellie and Ellen moved in with us. They were literally ready to leave the farm. Raised in rural Montana, they visited Grandma and Grandpa in Kansas City every summer and got a taste of big city life. In Kansas City, they knew they'd be welcomed by family and they could say goodbye to farm life forever.

Having Shellie and Ellen living with us was great for me and Jeremy too. Although Shellie was working, Ellen was going to cosmetology school and her schedule allowed her to pick up Jeremy from school and take care of him until I got home. It was a win-win all around!

One of the things my nieces and I loved to do together way sunbathe. Back in the early 1980s, we either didn't know or else ignored what hours of lying in the sun could do to your skin. Every chance we had, the girls and I sprawled out on lounge chairs in the yard to "work on our tan."

On one of those days, a tall, slim man wearing a cowboy hat stopped in front of us and asked if I could move my little Fiat convertible up a bit so he could park his eighteen-wheeler behind it. I sure could!

Turns out, the fellow was visiting my next-door neighbors who we were very friendly with. Jeremy and their son loved playing together.

That afternoon, my neighbor asked me to come by to "officially" meet her friend Brooks. I could tell very quickly that Brooks had his eye on me. The charisma, the flirting, it was pretty obvious. Brooks was the center of attention and put on a show. Jokes, stories, card tricks, the whole bonanza. He pulled out all the stops to impress me.

The next afternoon, Brooks asked if I'd like to go dancing with him. I accepted his kind offer. Brooks and I danced together like we'd been partners for years. I had a great time with him and vice versa.

The next weekend I took Jeremy on a trip out of town. When we got back, there was a dozen roses left at the neighbors' house because I was away. When Brooks found out I wasn't home, he was aggravated but I didn't think anything of it. At least in the beginning.

•

Like a twister goes through Kansas, I got swept up in the storm. Tornado Brooks. Yes, I was quite taken by all of the attention, the compliments, the conversations, and honestly, at first, his jealousy. I mean, here was someone who cared enough about me to be jealous. It was so different than feeling ignored by my ex David.

Like a love-struck teenager, I was lost in the whirlwind. As a result, after only a few months, I left my job and moved Jeremy to Colorado where Brooks had taken a job as a construction supervisor. Not only did I uproot my life but I was living with a man I wasn't married to…with my son. Jeremy's dad didn't like it, to say the least.

Back in 1984 when a woman moved in with a guy, child in tow, the courts did not take very kindly to it. Due to my fear that David might sue for custody of Jeremy, I decided to marry Brooks. It really had nothing to do with love. Very quickly, I learned a lot about my new husband. Things I should have tried to learn before uprooting Jeremy's and my life.

I soon got the feeling that Brooks was involved in some very shady business. An old friend of his was in charge of the construction job Brooks was hired on.

Almost immediately, I suspected that things weren't on the up and up. I could see there was criminal conduct going on involving stealing money, getting kickbacks and sneaking enough materials off the job site to build entire houses.

I'd never been around this kind of thing before. But my gut instinct told me that I shouldn't be anywhere near this sort of monkey business. It wasn't safe for me but more important, it wasn't safe for my son.

At first, pride stopped me from reaching out to my family and friends for help. I grew up in a very traditional home. Not only hadn't I'd ever seen anything like this before but I'd never met anyone like Brooks before. I was already divorced once and here I was, in another marriage on a collision course. It was embarrassing to admit that I'd screwed up yet again. I had no job, no savings plus Jeremy and I were a long way from home. I felt trapped.

The more I got to know the guys Brooks worked with—including his old buddy—the more jealous Brooks became. He thought I had designs on them and vice versa. Brooks and I could be out having a good time but when we got home, he'd be all over me, saying things like, "I saw that guy looking at your ass." As if it were MY fault.

Brooks had an irrational jealousy that got worse and worse the longer we were together. He wasn't physically abusive but he was scary jealous. There was the threat of violence behind his words. Brooks was exactly the kind of man who says, "If I can't have you no one can" and then does something rash. I believed Brooks could physically harm me, especially when he was drinking, which was often.

He had a mean streak you didn't want to be on the wrong side of. But fortunately, my husband's dirty dealings caught up with him.

•

When the FBI knocked on my door, I told them exactly where they could find Brooks and started packing. I thought/hoped I'd never see my husband again, which was fine with me.

Several hours later, Brooks came home spouting a fairy tale about how he was helping the Feds catch some bad dudes. His plan was to move us from Colorado to Florida where the developer of the Colorado project was based. Once we got there, Brooks swore that he'd be given a new position. At this point, I had trouble believing anything he said but I was ready to get far away from whatever was going down in Colorado. What I really wanted was a safe harbor for me and my son. But I didn't get it.

I don't think Jeremy realized how crazy this was at the time. He was so used to entertaining himself as an only child that Jeremy was very immersed in his own little world. But he might have been aware of some the nonsense going on, although I tried my best to shield him from it. As Jeremy got older, he certainly knew the score. But for the most part, I was able to make sure that Jeremy felt he and I were going to be alright.

It was important to me that my son knew he was the only person in the world I was concerned about. I made a promise to Jeremy that it was him and me, no matter what. Me and Jeremy against the world. That's when we started using an expression we used for the rest of his life: “It’s you and me ‘til the bitter end.”

Never did I think there WOULD be an end. And certainly not the bitter end that became a reality.

5

On the Move

Just after Jeremy and I moved to Florida with Brooks, my mother needed major surgery. Unfortunately, she had a stroke during the procedure. They ended up putting her on life support. This is not something my vibrant, outgoing mom would have wanted. I flew home and stayed for a couple weeks, sitting by her bedside, although she had no idea I was there.

The moment I saw my mother in the hospital bed, hooked up to tubes and buzzing machines, I knew her life was over. Until Jeremy and I moved to Colorado, I was very close to my mom. Losing her was a major, life-changing incident. Sadly, she didn't last very long in that debilitative state.

As I think back about it now, I don't even remember having the opportunity to grieve the loss of my mother. That's how deep I had sunk within my own chaos. I think my mom dying made me revert even further into isolation. She was the one who kept the family together. Without her, the entire family dynamic splintered and changed.

•

Of course, the Florida thing didn't pan out as Brooks had promised. When the money ran out, it was time to go. I flat out told Brooks that I'd called my old boss and explained my dire situation. My boss wired me money so Jeremy and I could get back to Kansas City. I didn't plan on ever seeing Brooks again. Or so I thought.

My son and I packed up what little we owned into a rented a U-Haul truck. Jeremy and I set out on the road, towing my Fiat behind us. It was starting to get dark when we got to the Florida/ Alabama state line. After paying the U-Haul rental, gas, and food, we didn't have much money left. Barely enough for a hotel. But I did something impulsive again.

My son's eyes lit up when he saw the signs for the Florabama fireworks store. I'd put him through so much moving him to Colorado, then Florida, then had uprooted him yet again. I figured the kid deserved a treat.

"Okay, here's the deal," I told Jeremy. "We can spend the money we have left on a motel room or we can sleep in the truck and spend the money on fireworks. It's up to you." What do you think my fun-loving kid chose?

To tell the truth, it really wasn't too uncomfortable sleeping in the truck, especially after watching

Jeremy have such a great time shopping for his big bag of fireworks.

The next day, he and I traveled on and midday, we stopped at a roadside diner for lunch. I couldn't believe my eyes when I looked up and saw Brooks coming through the door. He had actually found us on the road to Missouri! This made an indelible impression on me—Brooks must have been trailing us for hundreds of miles to "happen" upon us like that. I finally understood that Brooks wasn't going to let me go easy. It made me uncomfortable. And scared.

Finally arriving in Kansas City with Brooks tagging along, I realized that this relationship was not over. Far from it. I don't know why I couldn't make the break at the time, especially since I was back on my home turf where I had family and friends. But I believe that once again, it had a whole lot to do with pride mixed with an element of fear of how Brooks would react. Would he finally become physically violent? I knew it wasn't beyond him to publicly humiliate me with his dangerous jealousy. But what else was this man capable of?

•

I settled in as best I could and went back to work for my old boss. I was still bowled over by his generosity by sending money to help me out of a jam. Everything was going pretty smoothly until my workload increased and I had to spend a lot more time at work. The forty-five-minute commute each way was taking its toll on me. I hated spending so much time away from Jeremy but I also had to earn a living.

I don't remember what Brooks was doing for work during that time. He must have been doing something because I kept my money separate from his and I definitely wasn't supporting him. No doubt, it was something slightly illegal, knowing Brooks.

After about a year of being pulled apart in a tug of war from the demands of my job and Brooks' incessant and unrealistic jealousy, I woke up one morning, looked in the mirror and noticed that my right eyelid wasn't open. Did I have a stroke overnight?

I immediately made an appointment with a doctor, who thought it could be Turner Syndrome or even a possible brain tumor. Maybe it was nothing, he added, trying to ease my fears. I had a CT scan done on a Friday, which meant I would know nothing until at least Monday. Needless to say, I had an anxious weekend.

Thank God, the CT scan showed that my eye issue wasn't caused by anything in my brain. Eventually, the doctor narrowed it down to extremely high blood pressure. He put me on medication but in addition, wanted me to only work half days. As much of a saint as my boss was, he needed me full time. Reluctantly, I ended up leaving the job.

•

Without any prospects of generating an income until my health improved, I let Brooks talk me into moving to Arkansas where his family was. Besides there being a place for us to live, he had a building job lined up. I hoped that being close to his family, Brooks wouldn't drink as much. Maybe his crazy jealousy would be curbed too. I lived in hope. What else did I have?

Brooks did end up getting a job constructing a small motel for a couple who ran a fishing camp. Jeremy was able to do some work on the project, which gave him his first introduction to construction. My son soaked it up like a sponge and learned a lot. If one positive came out of our relationship, I'll credit Brooks with at least introducing Jeremy to something he loved.

The three of us lived in a very small town in the Arkansas mountains. It was a little too close to that movie *Deliverance* for my taste but I tolerated it. And Jeremy seemed to like it. When the construction project ended, Brooks took a job as a long-distance trucker. I was pleased because he was supposed to be gone for six weeks at a time. But of course, he couldn't stay away that long because Mr. Jealous needed to know what I was doing every moment.

On one of his trips away, I informed Brooks that I was going to look for a place to live closer to a large town. I managed to find a house ten miles from a good-sized city. It was a pretty area, out in the country, but at least it wasn't in the middle of nowhere.

When I put Jeremy in the sixth grade, I decided that I'd do everything I could to stay put until he finished school so he didn't have to move again.

In Jeremy's junior and senior years of high school, I went on the road with Brooks. I actually learned how to driving an eighteen-wheeler. Besides almost doubling the pay, Brooks figured he could monopolize my time and wouldn't be away from me at all. And me, I just liked the extra cash and the challenge of driving a semi.

While Brooks and I were on the road, Jeremy stayed home alone. I called him every night and he assured me he was fine. When I returned home after a few weeks, our next-door neighbor stopped by. I thought, *Oh Lord, what happened when I was gone? Girls, parties, what did he do?*

The neighbor lady began telling me that she and her husband were amazed that Jeremy was alone in the house and they never once saw anyone coming and going or any strange vehicles parked out front. Just him and his truck.

Growing up an only child, I guess Jeremy learned how to be alone. He didn't seem to mind as long as he had his computer, his pickup and his Commodore 128 (the latest home PC).

Jeremy graduated from high school in our Arkansas country town in 1993. He claimed he hardly ever opened a book and yet maintained an A average. Jeremy certainly was above average in intelligence and besides that, he was a go-getter. He got a job at Walmart when he was only sixteen.

After graduation, although Jeremy took classes at two different colleges, he decided college wasn't for him. He then opened a paintball field business. Although it didn't really make any money, it gave him and his friends a place to hang out and play paint ball. The business part of it allowed Jeremy to purchase the guns, paintballs and other equipment for himself. He traveled with a team to tournaments around the country and had some success at that.

I had every expectation that Jeremy would excel at whatever he did. Until the very end.

6

Charting a New Course

In 1994, Jeremy was grown and no longer needed my protection. In reality, at nineteen, he was old enough to protect me.

I made up my mind to get out of the relationship with Brooks once and for all. The opportunity presented itself clearly while we were away. A small electrical fire started in the house, and although there wasn't a lot of damage, the smoke and water had ruined most of my things. The insurance company had everything picked up by a restoration company so my furnishings were put into storage until I wanted them back.

There was a small bumper trailer that Jeremy had used at the paint ball field. He and I took our clothes, hitched up the trailer and took it to an RV park near Memphis, Tennessee. Brooks went his own way. With my husband finally out of the picture and my son and I living in a new place, I had to figure out a way to earn money.

•

Whenever I was in a casino, I'd always been fascinated watching dealers work the tables. The few times I'd been to Las Vegas, I played blackjack and enjoyed studying the dealers more than I enjoyed the "losing my money" part. I was captivated by the dealers, actually.

In 1990, gambling was legalized in Mississippi. So, by 1994 there were about six casinos in Tunica, which was approximately forty miles from Memphis. I set my sights on getting a job dealing cards. What did I have to lose?

Someone told me that one of the casinos was starting a class to teach prospective employees how to become dealers. It sounded perfect. But two weeks later, they cancelled the class and no one knew when or if there'd be another. I'm nothing if not resourceful. I was determined to learn on my own.

I started going to the casino every day. Without an "official" class to teach me, I simply stood back and watched the dealers' maneuvers at the blackjack tables. Since I couldn't afford to play, I studied the way they moved, where their hands were, how they handled the cards and how they dealt them out of a card "shoe"—a contraption which holds six decks.

Next, I went to the dollar store and bought a piece of felt which was very similar to the surface of a blackjack table. There, I also purchased several decks of cards and some play chips. When I came home after scrutinizing the dealers for a few hours,

I put my piece of felt on the trailer's little kitchen table and practiced dealing blackjack. Jeremy even pitched in, playing the part of my customer.

I knew that the only way to get a job dealing blackjack was to pass an audition. In it, you had to deal the game on a "live" table, with actual players and do it well enough to pass the critical eye of the pit boss standing behind you. No pressure! They didn't care where or how you learned to deal; they just cared that you actually possessed the skills required.

After a few weeks of watching and practicing, I felt like I might be able to do it. Circus Circus was the "break in" joint at that time. New dealers without experience were more likely to get hired there. Circus Circus handled small action, low bets, unlike the Horseshoe Casino next door, which was owned by Jack Binion. Jack's motto was, "There's no bet too big to take."

So, I figured it would be easier to get started at Circus Circus, which was known for taking on newcomers. I didn't think I was ready for the Horseshoe. Not yet.

I mustered my courage and made an appointment to audition. When the day arrived, I donned the dealer's "uniform"—a white shirt and black pants—and went to meet the pit boss. He took me behind the ropes and told the dealer to "tap out" so I could step in. I nearly said, "No, no, just kidding. I don't know how to do this." But somehow, I managed to steady my nerves.

As the dealer clapped her hands and stepped to the side, I found myself striding up to the table. It's all sort of a blur, but a few hands later, the pit boss had the dealer come back in and I clapped out. I'm pretty sure I was shaking. By some miracle—or maybe because they were desperate for dealers—I was hired!

Because Jeremy wasn't yet twenty-one, he couldn't get a job on a casino's gaming floor. He was, however, able to secure work in one of the casino hotels. Jeremy signed on as a customer service host, which meant he handled guest requests—things like gambling, dining and transportation. Sometimes he was even asked to arrange "dates" for high rollers.

Although he was under age, because Jeremy was 6' 2" and weighed in at two hundred and fifty pounds, he was never questioned as to his age when he visited another casino. That's where he started playing poker. Poker was something both he and I loved. This carried on throughout my career as a dealer and throughout the rest of his life.

My son and I toughed it out for a few months in the tiny trailer, taking showers in the RV park's bath house and living in close quarters. Before long, we were able to lease an apartment in a brand-new complex near work that was built with casino employees in mind. It would be great living closer to the job and would cut out a long commute each day. I could finally have my furniture brought out of storage and make a real home with my son.

•

Sometime in 1995, Brooks contacted Jeremy. I think he was trying to work his way back into my life by telling my son that he could get him in as

Assistant Superintendent on the construction project Brooks was currently working on in Memphis.

Now, that's not normally a position someone without an impressive construction resume could get. But Brooks' "gift" of being a convincing liar led the owner to believe that Jeremy had the experience needed for the position. The truth of the matter was that Jeremy didn't have the skills set when he took on the job. But he quickly learned how to read blueprints, do material take offs, and organize and schedule subcontractors. I don't think anyone doubted that Jeremy was experienced for a hot minute.

That's just one indication of how sharp and smart my son was. The construction job in Memphis actually ended up being serendipitous because when Brooks was fired from the job, Jeremy was made Superintendent. And that's how his twenty-year construction career was born!

My wonderful, protective son's departing words to Brooks were, "Don't ever contact my mom again!" And believe it or not, Brooks didn't.

7

True Friends Last a Lifetime

As Jeremy began to travel from state to state, building large apartment complexes and commercial buildings, the time we spent together was limited. So, I went from living with my son to seeing him only in the short space of days when one construction job ended and the next began. Although I spoke with Jeremy several times a week, it wasn't the same as seeing him in the flesh…hearing his infectious laugh, seeing him smile.

Over the next twenty years, Jeremy led construction projects in nine different states, the last twelve of those years in Louisiana. To give you a better idea of the kind of person my son was, I've asked two of his most important and influential friends to share some experiences they've had with Jeremy, both as a friend and as a business associate.

Early in Jeremy's career I met the man and woman who became Jeremy's best buddies. (You'll meet Linda, Jeremy's closest female friend, in the next chapter.) Harvey has impeccable ethics, a profound Christian belief system and a wonderful family. He's the kind of person who's a great judge of character and doesn't give praise without warrant.

Here's what Harvey had to say about my son Jeremy:

Harvey
"My Friend Jeremy"

"I first met Jeremy in the summer of 1995 in Memphis, Tennessee. I was working at an apartment complex doing clean-up and grading the soil around the buildings. Since the job was nearly complete, Jeremy was inside the structures themselves, doing what's called 'a punch out.' A punch out is a list of the minor things that need to be fixed before the contractor can turn it over to the owner. Jeremy was Assistant Superintendent on that job, second in command. Most of the contactors I'd worked with were standoffish with the 'clean-up crew' but Jeremy was different. He was just a happy twenty-year-old doing a job he enjoyed… and was good at.

"Jeremy and I hit it off right away. Maybe it was our mutual love for the outdoors or maybe it was just meant to be. But whatever the reason, I'm so grateful that in the summer of 1995, I made a friend for life that I would grow to love and deeply respect. Although we were always in contact, we didn't work on every job together. But whenever I did work with Jeremy, it was a treat.

"He and I took many hunting and fishing trips. We may not have gotten our quota of ducks or fish but one

thing was for sure—we always had a blast. In 2002, when Jeremy was working in Minot, North Dakota, he invited myself and a few friends to fly up for a goose and duck hunt. I told Jeremy that if he lined it up, I would cover his share of the expenses.

"In the end, it may have been less anxiety-producing to let Jeremy pay his own way but I insisted on treating him. After all, the six of us making this trip were being put up by Jeremy's girlfriend's family, so I figured the least I could do was pay his way, especially since they were hosting us, right?

"When we met the family, we were greeted by twenty pies sitting in the kitchen. I looked at Jeremy in disbelief. He just laughed and said, 'She's been cooking all week for you fellows.' I'm thinking, to hell with Daffy Duck. I don't want to hunt; I just want to eat these pies!"

"Let me tell you, we had an absolute blast the next six days. When the week came to a close and we had to fly back south, we thanked our wonderful hosts and headed to the airport. As I shared the ride with Jeremy, he said, 'Harvey, I really appreciate you paying my way.' And dropped it. I immediately knew he was up to something because normally we'd have a thirty-minute argument with him handing me money and me handing it back.

"We arrived at the airport about three hours before our flight and checked all the bags except our carry-ons. On the way, we'd spotted a sporting goods store nearby so we decided to walk over there to kill some time. After all, we were seven hunters! We couldn't resist.

"When we passed Jeremy's truck, he said, 'Come here, Harvey, I want to give you something.' He

reached into the truck and pulled out a brand-new Sig 45 pistol. Jeremy explained, 'I know you won't take money for the trip but I really want you to have this.'

"I stopped for a second and said, 'Jeremy, I'm really grateful for this and I want you to know that if you ever need or want it back, it's yours.' I still have that gun to this very day.

"After Jeremy gave me the pistol, I put it in my backpack and caught up with the other guys. Tim, one of the fellows in the group, bought a 'handy tool' at the sporting goods store.

"Back at the airport, we said our goodbyes to Jeremy and the rest of us headed to the TSA security check. Now, mind you, this was the fall of 2002, just a year after the World Trade Center disaster, so airport security was pretty tight. Tim put his backpack on the conveyor belt and I pitched mine next to his.

"We passed through the x-ray machine without problem but one bag didn't. A TSA agent pointed to Tim's backpack and asked, 'Whose bag is this?' Turns out the tool he'd bought had a four-inch knife blade in it. They nicely asked him to throw it away and he did.

"I reached for my backpack and headed to the plane just as it started boarding. I put my pack in the overhead compartment and settled in for the long flight. My buddy Jason was sitting behind me. He tapped me on the shoulder and asked, 'Where is that 45?'

"I thought, Holy crap! but calmly said to Jason, 'It's just above your head.'

"'What are you going to do?' Jason asked.

"'I said, 'I'm going to change planes in Minneapolis and fly home.' Jason gave me a wide-eyed look but didn't say another word about it.

"We landed in Minneapolis and had a four-hour layover. All the while, I was tightly gripping the backpack containing the 45. We boarded the plane for the last leg of our trip, landed in Memphis and were relieved that my weapon hadn't been discovered.

"Later I told Jeremy the story and we had a good laugh over it. 'Thanks, Jeremy,' I told him. 'But next time you want to give me a gun, let's consider shipping it.' The headline could have been, 'Home-Grown Terrorists Smuggle Weapons Onboard Plane!' But thankfully, we weren't put on the 'no fly' list.

"The next year, in the summer of 2003, Jeremy and I were working together on a project in Arkansas. My parents moved their fifth-wheel trailer there so they could live in comfort while my dad ran my crew. Jeremy was the Superintendent on the job site and I was glad because I knew he'd look after my folks while they were there. I was finishing up a job in Kentucky and would be onsite in Arkansas as soon as possible.

"One day, I got a phone call from Jeremy saying, 'We have a little problem.' My heart dropped when I asked what happened. Jeremy explained that my dad had run a Bobcat (a small excavator machine that landscapers use) into one of the finished apartment buildings. But thank God my pop wasn't hurt.

"I asked Jeremy what my dad said and Jeremy replied, 'Mr. Jack came into my office and said 'Jeremy, you and Harvey have some mess to clean up.' Then he retired to his trailer for the day. Jeremy could have made a big deal about this but he didn't. He simply took it in stride. My dad loved Jeremy like a son and Jeremy always took care of and respected Mr. Jack and my mom. I loved Jeremy all the more for that.

"Sometime later, Jeremy was starting a job in Lafayette, Louisiana and wanted me to take the landscaping contract. He said he needed someone 'good,' and that was me. After Jeremy sent me the blueprints, we hashed out the job details and the cost. I signed on and looked forward to working with Jeremy in Lafayette.

"But what he failed to mention was that the dirt work was over a crawfish farm and the mosquitoes were the size of new-hatched sparrows. A minor detail.

"After the buildings went up, I went to the Lafayette jobsite. The complex was next to a golf course, so in the afternoons I walked the property picking up the golf balls that had landed there. Some of them even broke windows but we didn't make a fuss about it.

"Late one evening, just as I finished up my daily ritual and was getting into my truck with a five-gallon bucket full of golf balls, I saw a white golf cart speeding down the street. It was driven by a dark-skinned man dressed in all white clothing. The fellow pulled up to my truck and motioned for me to roll down my window. When I did, in a very heavy Jamaican accent, the guy started screaming, 'I want my balls! I want my balls!' over and over.

"I said to him, 'I don't think I've ever seen your balls!'

"He didn't appreciate the humor because he shouted back, 'No, I want my golf balls!' Right then, it hit me that Jeremy was inside the office trailer, listening to this whole exchange and laughing his butt off.

"I said to the angry man, 'If you want your balls, follow me.' I knew I could get to Jeremy before the 'ball guy' could.

"When I walked into the trailer, Jeremy nonchalantly said, 'What's up?' though he knew full well what was up.

"I said, 'This nice man wants to talk to you.' As Ball Guy walked through the door, I pulled up a chair to watch the show. On cue, the door burst open and the man screamed, 'I want my balls!' Jeremy looked at me helplessly.

"I shrugged and said, 'Man, I'm just the landscaper' as Ball Guy continued ranting.

"Now, Jeremy had a very long fuse; he was the most non-confrontational Superintendent I'd ever met. But, once this fuse was lit, the best thing to do was to get out of the way of this massive teddy bear. Jeremy stood up and said, 'Sir, get your butt out of my office and off my property. If your clients keep breaking my windows with your balls, I'll put your balls in jail!' Ball Guy was speechless but left quietly.

"Another time, when Jeremy and I were on the same project in Cleveland, Tennessee, he texted and asked me to come to his trailer. When I walked in, Jeremy starting making small talk. After a couple minutes, he said, 'I have a problem on the property and I don't know what to do about it.' I knew Jeremy was setting me up to come to the rescue but I respected the fact that he thought enough of me to ask for help.

"Jeremy proceeded to explain that the building specs called for a retainer wall to be built behind a building on the contour of the property. So, I'm thinking, Okay…and? Jeremy went on to say that the church next door was going to build an eight-foot fence on the property line that would prevent us from putting up our retainer wall. Then the clincher! 'We've got two days to get it done and it's going to start snowing soon!'

"I asked Jeremy, 'Do you have money in the budget for this wall?'

"He answered, 'All we need.' My reply was simply to order two light trailers to help us along. He did and we worked through the night. By the next morning, the wall was finished. Jeremy bought me breakfast and smiled, 'See, I knew you could do it.'

"My last job with Jeremy was in 2012 to 2013, again in Lafayette, Louisiana. It turned out absolutely beautiful. No problems, no stress. Jeremy was the best Project Manager I ever worked for.

"As I think back over the more than twenty years I knew Jeremy, we never had a harsh word or an argument. I truly cherish the friendship I had with Jeremy and I miss him every day.

"The last time I saw Jeremy was March 2018. I noticed that he had lost a lot of weight but when I asked him about it, he said, 'I've been dieting.'

"I'll never forget where I was when I found out Jeremy was gone. I was hunting on a mountain in Idaho when my wife called and sobbed, 'We've lost Jeremy!'

"I said, 'Jeremy who?' It was a complete and total shock to me that he could be gone. Then I found out how it happened and I felt even more terrible. I felt like I had let Jeremy down because I should have seen the signs. I should have been a better friend. I should have helped him but I had no clue.

"I moved from those emotions to being totally pissed off at Jeremy. I walked around mad at him for weeks. I remember thinking, You idiot! You hurt so many people who loved and needed you!

"After a while I realized that if Jeremy could have changed things, he would have. Now I just remember

all the good times we shared and how he made me a better man. And that's a lot."

8

True Friends Last a Lifetime
Part Two

The woman who became Jeremy's closest female friend had a star-crossed love affair with him for more than twenty years. These are some memories Linda shared with me after Jeremy's death. I'm very grateful that she did. It gave me so much more insight about my son.

Lovely, Lonely Linda
"JJ"
"RACEN4LUV"

"Jeremy came into my life in an unusual way. Maybe it was meant for us to meet. I was twenty-eight years old, married and so lonely. My husband had just accepted a new job in another state and left me to take care of our two small children, age three and five. At the same time, I also had to deal with moving away from the only home I'd ever known. This meant moving

away from my family. It was a lot to deal with emotionally.

"In my solitude, I started looking for things to occupy myself. Around 1996, America Online (AOL) had become a 'thing.' Besides being an email platform, it was probably the first people-connecting platform created. There were 'chat rooms' where you could 'enter' and make connections, meet new friends with similar interests and interact with people all over the world. At the time, it was very innovative and cutting edge.

"I 'met' Jeremy in an AOL chat room in 1995. We shared a love of NASCAR and all things racing. My AOL 'handle' was 'LuvRacin2.' I found myself in a chat room called 'Ask a Male Anything.' That's where I first saw the name 'RACEN4LUV' which was Jeremy's AOL 'handle.' I was intrigued.

"My main reason for being in the chat room was to find out if guys cheated on their significant other when they were in a different zip code, knowing they could get away with it because of the miles that separated them. 'RACEN4LUV' jumped in and immediately started answering my questions. Later, he said it was because he liked my ID name. He also said that he was twenty-five. Being naïve, I believed him!

"Right off the bat, RACE seemed so genuinely sweet. He asked to exchange pictures so we did. It seemed innocent enough. The guy in the picture would turn out to be my best friend, my 'person,' my soulmate.

"RACE and I went online and talked for as long as we could before life interrupted us. Eventually, I gave him my phone number. Whenever he called, we chatted for hours late into the night. Our phone calls stopped when my kids and I joined my husband in North Carolina.

"When I got to the Carolinas, I was still alone. My husband was very engrossed in his new job and his new friends. I went back online but couldn't find 'RACEN4LUV.' I can't say I wasn't disappointed. Oh well, I thought, It was fun while it lasted.

"To fill the void, I decided to become an AOL guide. Guides were there to jump from chat room to chat room and make sure everyone was 'behaving.' Then I saw him! RACE and I started talking again and it was great. At this point, I knew I needed to meet him in person, so we made plans to meet in Tampa where I was going to visit a friend.

"I was so nervous on that flight. Would I be able to pick RACE out of a crowd? The minute I stepped into the airport, there was Jeremy waiting for me. Oh, those dimples… I knew it was him immediately.

"Jeremy and I hugged like we had known each other for years instead of just months online. He felt was warm and safe, like my childhood teddy bear. We spent three wonderful days getting to know each other and sharing our life stories.

"That's when Jeremy came clean about his real age. He was actually twenty-one, not twenty-five. In the next breath, he told me that he loved me. I was flattered but said, 'I'm too old for you; I'm twenty-eight. Besides, I'm married and have two little kids!' It seemed like the smart thing to say at the time. But I have to admit I had very strong feelings for Jeremy.

"A few weeks passed without us having any contact with each other. I suddenly realized how much I missed our conversations, his warmth and the comfort I felt when I was with him. But as tough as it was, I didn't waiver on whether or not I should have a relationship with Jeremy. Just like I'd explained to him, I was

married with two young children. But truthfully, I missed Jeremy like I missed a best friend, and more.

"My life changed drastically in July 1996. A lady I'd met only once came to my house and told me that my husband was cheating on me with a woman they both worked with. I had a gut feeling something was going on because he was rarely home. But I ignored my instincts until this woman confirmed my fears. I guess in order to survive, I pretended it wasn't happening. But then someone put it in front of my face!

"What was I going to do? I was in a new place with no friends, no job and two young kids. I was lost, confused and hurt. I had no one to turn to. No one except Jeremy. He listened patiently to my tale of woe then told me to put the children in the car and come to Memphis. So, that's exactly what I did!

"Jeremy and I shared another few days together. It was great. He got along well with my kids too. He wanted us to stay with him in Memphis. But how could I? He was still only twenty-two by then. True, he had a good job but how could I burden him with supporting me and my two little ones? I didn't think it was fair to him so I returned to North Carolina.

"I missed Jeremy so much! I couldn't wait to see him again. Along with a couple of our AOL friends, we planned a party for August at my house. We invited a bunch of our other online friends. We thought it would be epic and it was. Everyone came. We had a blast!

"Even my husband joined in the festivities. Until he took it to a whole other level. I woke up in the middle of the night to find him having sex with one of my AOL 'friends.' Right there in our home! I was so upset and humiliated that I woke Jeremy. He actually 'outed' them by turning on the light for all to see. Talk about

humiliation! I asked my husband and my former online friend to leave. Jeremy held me in his arms the rest of the night, not saying a word.

"After a couple of weeks, Jeremy came to visit me in North Carolina. That's when I asked him to stay. He said he would. But between that visit and his moving into my home, Hurricane Fran happened. In September 1996, most of my area flooded so I had no power, no supplies and no help since my husband was staying elsewhere.

"I was shocked when my estranged husband came back to the house to help in the aftermath of Hurricane Fran. I was so desperate, I let him. He begged for forgiveness and wanted to come home. I told him that I'd asked Jeremy to move into the spare bedroom. To my surprise, my husband had no problem with that.

"So, Jeremy came to stay for a couple of months. He'd completed the construction project he was on so there was a lull until his next one started. As a temporary job, he actually started selling cars in North Carolina. I felt so lucky to have my best friend with me every day but I was also conflicted. Could I really leave my husband to be with Jeremy? I didn't have to make that difficult decision because Jeremy soon left to take a job in Tennessee.

"Our next adventure was in May 1998. Jeremy and I went to Savannah, Georgia to another gathering of AOL friends, this time, on a camping trip. No husband, no kids, no worries! Jeremy and I knew without a doubt that we were in love with each other. But there was nothing we could do about it because I was still tied to my husband. So, Jeremy and I vowed to see each other whenever we could.

"Soon after, Jeremy left for his job in Tennessee. When school ended, I took my kids to Connecticut to visit family. Jeremy came to visit me up there. Over the next year, I also went to see Jeremy in Tennessee. Then, we spent five days in Las Vegas and later, met up in Philadelphia. Our long-distance love affair was unbreakable.

"At the end of 1999, my husband was transferred to Arizona. Since I was finally working and making money of my own, I told him that I didn't want to go. He said there was no other option. Either I went with him or he'd take the kids and leave without me. So, on January 4, 2000, my family and I left North Carolina.

"By that point, Jeremy was frustrated with me. He thought I should stand up for myself in my marriage and demand what I wanted instead of constantly caving in to my husband's whims. But despite his frustrations with me, Jeremy came to see me in Arizona that March. Again, we had a wonderful time.

"A few months later, Jeremy and I met up in Modesto, California. That's when Jeremy told me that he wanted to start seeing other people. He was looking for a serious relationship and I was unavailable. Although it crushed me, I actually encouraged Jeremy to do it. Our long-distance relationship wasn't fair to him. Understandably, we started to drift apart.

"Reluctantly, I went on with my life. I returned to college to finish my degree, got a new job, built my career and raised my kids. Jeremy was busy navigating a very successful construction career. We talked occasionally throughout those next seven years. The love was most definitely still there but making a life-changing choice would affect many others, especially my children, so once again, I couldn't commit to Jeremy.

"In 2008, it happened again: my husband cheated on me. The very same man who had begged for forgiveness, moved the family across country time and again, the very same man I stayed with instead of building a life with my soulmate, Jeremy. This time, I knew my marriage was over. My kids were teenagers, I was completing my Master's degree and I could finally make it on my own. So, we separated again and this time, I went through with the divorce.

"As I still did occasionally, I called Jeremy. I filled him in on my latest news and asked him if perhaps we could give us a real try, this time without the complication of my marriage getting in the way. That's when Jeremy told me that he'd met someone. Jeremy was going to get married! She had a one-year-old girl and a two-and-a-half-year-old boy. The kids' father was out of the picture. Jeremy had fallen in love—with them and her.

"Although I was happy for him, I was also devastated. This could have been me! This could have been my kids. For twelve years, I was in love with Jeremy but I kept making excuses about why I shouldn't be with him. Now I had the opportunity to try and make it work with him and he'd finally found someone else.

"As I moved on, I never stopped caring about Jeremy, even after his marriage. I got into a new relationship and ended up getting married on the rebound. I was miserable almost immediately but my stubbornness forced me to stick with my commitment. I moved back to Connecticut in 2010 with my new husband John and tried to make it work.

"For the first couple of years I was happy, or at least I tried to convince myself that I was. Then in

2013, I got a call from Jeremy. He told me his wife had cheated on him with a woman and he was done. We talked about the kids he was raising with her. He explained to me that he'd made a commitment to those children, regardless of what their mother did. He was going to raise them as his own. He would always be their dad, he said.

"I had so much respect for him! But again, this was a blow to my heart. Maybe I should have waited for Jeremy but I couldn't. I had to fill the void somehow so I rushed into a bad marriage. What wounded me the most about Jeremy's current situation was knowing how badly he was hurting. We continued to talk while he was going through his divorce but I was married again so Jeremy and I didn't resume our affair.

"In 2013, a job transfer brought me back to Arizona. Jeremy called and said he happened to be going to Arizona on a gold mining vacation with his father. I really wanted to see Jeremy but did I want to go down that road again? It was a tough choice but I didn't end up seeing him. I was still hurt by the fact that he chose get married instead of giving us a real shot.

"As fate would have it, Jeremy and I discovered that we'd both be in Colorado at the same time. I missed him and didn't want to miss this chance. My life now consisted of playing nursemaid to a husband who wouldn't help himself. John was just looking for a caretaker, not a life partner.

"At that point, I just felt defeated. I needed Jeremy! I needed his warmth, his love, his voice of reason in my head. So, I went to Colorado to see him. We spent several days together visiting some of the most beautiful places in the state. Plus, he introduced me to his dad.

"I was so happy during those few days in Colorado. It was as if no time had passed since we'd last seen each other. Just like every other time. I shared with Jeremy everything that had happened since I'd been back in Arizona and how I regretted my decision to get married. I also told him how hurt I'd been that he got married when we could have finally been together in a committed relationship. This upset him. So much so that we actually had our first argument in eighteen years. Later that night, he and I laughed about having our first spat but it still wounded him that I was married.

"Jeremy and I saw each other again in December of that year when I had to travel to Mississippi for work. Jeremy was nearby in Louisiana so I extended my trip for a day and drove to one state over to visit him. We spent a wonderful twenty-four hours together there. He showed me his office and the other jobs he'd completed in Lafayette.

"When I returned to Arizona, I decided once and for all that I wanted out of my marriage. I applied for a new position in Florida—and got it. I told my husband John that I wanted a divorce and left for the Sunshine State.

"In August 2015, Jeremy came to visit me in my temporary Florida digs. We went to a couple of escape rooms, something I'd never heard of before he told me about them. If you've never heard of them, an escape room is a type of interactive game where a team of players discover clues, solve puzzles and perform tasks in order to get out of a room or series of rooms within a set amount of time. Visiting escape rooms was a lot of fun, especially with Jeremy.

"When he told me that he wanted to create, build and open an escape room business in Louisiana, I was

so happy for him. But on the romance front, I couldn't for the life of me figure out how we'd be able to keep up a long-distance relationship. But we swore we'd try.

"A couple months later, John withdrew the divorce petition in Arizona, drove to Florida and pleaded with me to take him back. I can't explain why I did it other than I felt sorry for him. But I took John back. Against my better judgement, I took him back.

"Once more, Jeremy was disappointed in me. It was the first time I actually felt like he didn't care about me. He totally withdrew from me, that's how hurt he was. I wanted him to succeed and build his creative dream. And he did! I was so proud of him!

"Time passed and somehow, it was 2018. Once again, I was going to be relocated, this time back to North Carolina. Nostalgia got the best of me because on the day after my birthday, I called Jeremy—since he didn't, for the first time in more than twenty years, call me on my birthday. I told him I was moving back to North Carolina and that I was still miserable in my marriage. Jeremy seemed different that day. I could tell he wasn't happy but he apologized for missing my birthday. I just knew something was off but I couldn't tell what.

"A little while later, Jeremy called asking for money. He said the business wasn't doing well and he needed help to make payroll. I thought this was strange because I was following him and the Escape Room on social media and things seemed to be going great.

"When I got to Charlotte, I called Jeremy and asked if he'd come visit since I was in temporary housing. Alone. That moment my world changed! He told me the truth about what had been going on with him over the past several months: drugs, arrests, deep

disappointment in himself. That's why Jeremy couldn't leave the state to come see me.

"At first, I didn't believe him. This had to be a bad joke. How could this beautiful soul have turned to drugs and associate himself with those kinds of people? I just couldn't understand it. I did what I could from a moral support perspective and told Jeremy that I'd come see him as soon as possible. Most likely, it would be after Thanksgiving, after I settled into my new job and new home.

"My final visit with Jeremy came sooner than I'd expected. But it wasn't anything I could ever have imagined.

"My last phone conversation with Jeremy was on October 12· 2018. He was upbeat and said he was looking forward to the Kansas City Chiefs playing the New England Patriots on Sunday night football. This was our personal rival game, since I was a New Englander and he was born in Kansas City. When Jeremy didn't text me during the game, I thought something was up. But he knew I was traveling to Ohio on business and so I figured that's why he didn't reach out to me.

"On Monday evening, I received the worst news of my life. A call came in from Jeremy's cell phone number but it wasn't him on the other end of the line. It was Jeremy's mom telling me that he was gone. I will never forget that feeling for the rest of my life. It was like the bottom dropped out of me.

"All of the what ifs in the world can't explain the whys. While Jeremy and I were never able to have our happy ending, his death has empowered me. I helped me grow to be a strong independent woman who refuses to live by any rules other than her own. I

have given myself permission to be happy and I vow to walk away when I'm not. Plus, I now have a dear, new friend—Jeremy's mother Carol.

"For twenty-two years during Jeremy's life and for the rest of mine, I will love him. Jeremy was my 'person,' my soulmate, my best friend. I am forever grateful for this and I will never take another day for granted."

9

Life Takes Its Course

Jeremy settled into his construction career and found his passion. Over the course of his profession, he built numerous commercial projects, multi-family housing, student housing and senior housing throughout the United States, including Tennessee, Arkansas, Mississippi, Kentucky, Florida, North Dakota, Nebraska, Alabama and Louisiana.

My son made friends everywhere he went. While working in North Dakota in 2002, he met a very nice girl named Jackie. She traveled with him and lived with him for the next four years. Jackie and Jeremy made a great couple but it ultimately came down to her wanting to start a family and him not being ready for it.

When they broke up, they packed Jackie up and put her belongings into the small U-Haul trailer Jeremy rented. He drove her back to North Dakota without much ceremony. But I know Jeremy felt bad about it because he still had feelings for Jackie. He continued to support her for a few months until she found a job and got back on her feet. Jeremy was kindhearted in every way.

•

As for me, after about two years of dealing blackjack, I had the opportunity to meet one of the pit bosses at the Horseshoe Casino. At that time, you actually had to be "juiced in," as they called it. This meant that you had to know somebody to even get an audition there.

The big difference between Circus Circus and the Horseshoe? Money! Dealers at the Horseshoe were making about three times the amount in tips as dealers at Circus Circus.

Without the case of the jitters I'd had when I tried out at Circus Circus, I passed my audition at the Horseshoe with flying colors. I'd learned a lot and was skilled enough to pass muster at this high-end, high-rollers' casino. After the audition, the pit told me, "Gee, I finally can recommend someone who's actually an excellent dealer."

I loved it there! The Horseshoe was the place where any "star" who traveled through the area stopped to gamble. In the late 1990s, celebrities like comedian Dick Cavett, country singer George Jones, golfer John Davidson and basketball great Michael Jordan came into the Horseshoe. It was always a kick to watch the top-shelf treatment they received.

•

When Jeremy came home to visit and had a few days off, he would play poker. Although I had grown up playing the game, you didn't find many women at the tables other than the dealers. I started playing in the casinos when Jeremy did and soon, I was a regular.

My son and I both loved poker tournaments so he tried to be home to take part in them whenever he could. When Jeremy was working in North Dakota, he actually won the Dakota Jim Dandy Poker Festival, which had a $10,000 prize. It was televised on one of the local TV channels and he even made me a tape of it so I could watch him play.

Teasing Jeremy, I often told him, "When I die, I want you to take $10,000 of my insurance money and play in the World Series of Poker Main Event." The biggest poker tournament in the world, the Main Event was held in Las Vegas every year. Jeremy and I watched it on TV every year, so it would be a milestone to play in that event.

By 1997, I was no longer enamored with dealing blackjack so I wanted to transition to dealing poker. Poker was in a completely separate department than the casino's other games so this would be a big move. But just like blackjack, I learned how to deal poker from playing it and again, by practicing on my own.

Although I knew there were a couple of openings in the poker department, I waited several months to ask for a transfer. I also knew there was a waiting list of people trying to get a job in the poker room.

Finally, one day I met the poker room manager in the back of the house and said to him, "I know you're looking to hire dealers and I already work here dealing black jack, so don't you think I should have first shot at the job?" He agreed and set up an audition for me soon after. When I went to my poker audition, I knew almost everyone playing and dealing in the room, so that made it easy for me. I got my transfer and my dream job!

•

I had been visiting Biloxi, Mississippi for several years playing poker in its casinos and seeing friends there. It was a beautiful area. Because the Gulf Coast and the Mississippi River converge in Louisiana, you had two totally different environments and vibes. There were twenty-five miles of manmade beach. I fell instantly in love!

So, in 1999, when the Beau Rivage Casino was set to open, I decided to move to Biloxi and try to get a job dealing poker there since they'd be needing more dealers in the new place. Unfortunately, the poker room at the Beau closed just four months after opening, so there were a lot of experienced dealers looking for a job besides me.

Although I was unable to get a job dealing poker, I took a pit boss job at another casino. Boring! But at least my divorce with Brooks was finalized while I was there, so that was good.

I worked at the Beau for about nine months when I called my old boss at the Horseshoe back up in Tunica to ask if I could "come home."

"Of course," he said.

So, I packed up, relocated to Tunica and went back to the Horseshoe.

On my time off, I played poker at several of the casinos, especially The Grand. It was at the Grand that I met Gerald. He was a dealer on the late shift and was always very sweet but quiet. But I kind of liked that.

All of the dealers who played poker played at the various casino rooms in the area. I played at the Grand, Gerald played at the Horseshoe and we both played at Circus Circus. As he and I became better acquainted, I realized that Gerald was a kind and gentle soul. Almost too good to be true after what I'd been through with other men. We started dating and I don't think we were ever apart after our second date.

Gerald and I moved in together and basically worked the same schedule at different casinos. Jeremy knew Gerald from playing poker with him many times and my son was happy to hear we were together. I was glad that Gerald liked Jeremy too.

My beau and I continued to live in the Tunica area until 2002. That year, the tables at the Grand Casino poker room were extremely slow. Since the majority of dealers' income came from tips, this was a big blow financially. Gerald was only making half of what he normally did.

About that time, I heard that the Grand Casino in Biloxi was hiring poker dealers. I'd made friends with lots of the dealers and management when I was living there, so I called a fellow named John and asked if Gerald and I could come down and audition for a job. John welcomed that idea.

The next string of days Gerald and I had off, we drove the three-hundred-and-fifty miles to Biloxi and met with John. Gerald and I had an audition with about eight other dealers who were also seeking jobs there. When we finished, John asked me into his office. He said, "You're good. I guess you and Gerald come as a package?"

"Yeah," I said, "That's kind of the way it is."

"Don't get me wrong," John told me. "Gerald's a good dealer, he's just really quiet."

I explained that Gerald was probably a little nervous, having never met John before. He'd also never been in that poker room before. But I assured John that Gerald would be great at the job and the customers would love him. And they did.

Both Gerald and I were hired at the Grand Casino. We returned to Tunica, gave a two weeks' notice and set to move to Biloxi. You never want to burn a bridge in that business—it's so small and insular and everyone knows everyone else—so we made our exit from Tunica the right way. We found a place to live in Biloxi, arranged for a truck and arrived there a little over two weeks later, ready to roll.

10

Tumultuous Years

Not long after our move to Biloxi, Gerald and I decided to get married. We wanted to buy a house to retire in, not to mention we were very much in love. Gerald was one of the most wonderful men I've ever known. Kind, sweet and thoughtful, he had a beautiful singing voice and a great ear besides. He would hear a song once, know the words and sing it back perfectly.

Gerald and I made plans to have a small, simple wedding with just a few people present. I called Jeremy, who was working in Tennessee at the time. I asked if he and Jackie would be our witnesses. (Yes, Jeremy was still with Jackie at that point.) They were thrilled and honored we'd asked and of course, agreed.

On September 19, 2003, Gerald and I were married in the gazebo at Biloxi City Park. A judge did the honors and Jeremy and Jackie were our witnesses. My co-workers held a small wedding reception for us at a bar near the casino. It was very nice.

Less than two years later, that beautiful gazebo would be destroyed by Hurricane Katrina. A memorial stands in its place to honor the fifty-three people from Biloxi who lost their lives in that storm. But on a lovely September day in 2003, that gazebo was filled with joy.

•

Next on my new husband and my agenda was finding a permanent home. We wanted somewhere to set down roots and eventually, retire in. A coworker mentioned that she'd had her house built in a pretty, new development in Ocean Springs. The Ocean Springs neighborhood was a terrific community. It's just across a bridge from Biloxi so it was an excellent location too. The downtown area is an artsy, foodie, touristy kind of place that offers a wide variety of entertainment options. It sounded perfect.

Gerald and I decided to take a look at the newest subdivision being built in Ocean Springs. It was a "cookie cutter" sort of neighborhood with five or six different housing style options. But the buyer was able to select some of the finishes at the base price, personalizing their home exactly the way they wanted to.

We met the realtor representing the developer and he took us to see the remaining lots available. Although there weren't many left, we managed to find one we liked. The house could be set back in the middle of the lot and still leave plenty of room for a front yard, side yard and backyard. Gerald and

I picked the floorplan we wanted and started the exciting process of having our retirement home built.

It felt good to be planning ahead for life after work even though I was only fifty-four and Gerald was only fifty-two. Because he had no children and Jeremy was my "only," my son would handle our estate after Gerald and I passed. Because of this, we deeded the house to Jeremy so he wouldn't have any legal hassles regarding the house when my husband and I were no more.

Gerald and I moved into our home in March 2004. We loved every bit of it.

•

In the winter of that very same year, Gerald was dealing poker one day when the pit boss came to me and said, "Go look at Gerald and see if he's okay."

"Why?" I asked.

"A player just told me that Gerald sort of spaced out while he was dealing and he was kind of out of it for a minute."

I hurried over to the table where Gerald was working and watched him for a few moments. Something was clearly wrong. I told the boss to get Gerald out of his chair so we could see what was going on. My husband was definitely exhibiting strange symptoms. He was confused, shaky and his color was horrible.

After sitting for a while, Gerald said he felt fine and could drive himself home. A doctor's appointment was certainly in order. Gerald was diabetic but these weren't the usual symptoms associated with blood sugar issues. His doctor ran a series of tests to get to the bottom of the cause. It definitely wasn't connected to Gerald's diabetes and since he was never a smoker or a drinker, there was no obvious answer.

Some of Gerald's symptoms mimicked hepatitis but every test for hepatitis was negative. After about eight months of trying different drugs with moderate success, the doctor said that he wanted to do a liver biopsy to see if Gerald's condition might be autoimmune hepatitis. A liver biopsy is very painful but it seemed to be the only diagnostic option. Gerald had the biopsy.

Sure enough, a few days later, the biopsy confirmed the doctor's suspicion of autoimmune hepatitis. The disease can cause a build-up of ammonia in the body which can result in confusion and balance issues. Gerald continued to work as much as he could but sometimes it was difficult with the fatigue and discomfort he experienced.

Then, in the summer of 2005, I needed cataract surgery. They typically do one eye at a time with about two weeks between procedures. I had to wear a patch overnight and then return to check in with doctor the following day. He was very pleased with the results and I was too. I could finally see clearly!

But unfortunately, my second surgery didn't go so well.

You see, in cataract surgery, material behind the eye is dislodged during the procedure but it normally clears up quickly. However, mine didn't. The result? I wasn't able to see anything out of my right eye. I was blind in one eye!

For the next two weeks, I saw the doctor every few days to check if my eye material had been reabsorbed as she'd hoped. But no such luck. We had never discussed what might happen if the surgery failed. And I didn't want to know.

Although the complications from my cataract surgery was a left hook I wasn't expecting, there was more to come. August 29, 2005 changed everything!

•

Living on the Gulf of Mexico, we were used to hurricane warnings and even evacuations. The Mississippi Gaming Commission makes the call on whether the casinos will close when a hurricane is headed for the area. Of course, the casino operators don't want to close their doors for any reason but the final word comes from the Commission.

Whenever a hurricane was upon us, the management waited until the very last hour to get everyone out so security could come in and remove all the money and chips to an offsite location. In the last two years, we'd done two evacuations. The normal procedure was for the employees to drive five hours north to Tunica and stay at one of the casinos there.

You could only imagine the "hurricane parties" that went on. Gambling and carousing with fellow workers were a blast. The bad part was that the next day we were usually called back to work at our regularly-scheduled time to re-open the casino in Biloxi. So, we made the five-hour drive home then went to work in the evening.

Only Thursday, August 25, 2005 was different. The poker room at the Grand was crowded as usual. But instead of the many televisions in the room being tuned to sports channels, they were all playing the Weather Channel. This was an oddity. It should have alerted us as to the severity of the storm.

Casinos actually do things to isolate customers from the outside world. If you go to a gaming establishment, you'll notice that there are no clocks and very few windows. Most of the TVs play some kind of entertainment, mostly sports. They do this on purpose so you lose your frame of reference and all sense of time. You might not know if it's night or day, rainy or sunny. So, for all the TV screens to be tuned to the weather, you knew something was brewing.

Both employees and players began glancing up at the storm updates. A huge hurricane was growing over the Gulf and it was getting bigger and badder by the hour.

Everyone began relating their hurricane experiences as most of them had lived in this storm-prone area for decades. Stories traveled about Hurricane Camille. As I recall, it was the second most intense hurricane ever reported and one of only five Category 5 hurricanes to make landfall in the US. Camille hit Biloxi on August 17, 1969 and devastated real estate along the Mississippi coast. Several memorials serve as reminders of that storm.

Lots of people bragged about having hurricane parties and boasted about how many hurricane warnings they'd ignored to ride out the storm. Some saw it as a badge of honor to defy nature and hold their ground. Others saw it as just plain foolish.

Jeremy was living and working in Tuscaloosa, Alabama at that time. When a hurricane was headed my way, he and I were in frequent contact about the storm. Always concerned about Gerald's and my safety, Jeremy was constantly considering every possible evacuation plan for us. It meant a lot to me how much my son worried about me plus I was in awe of how pragmatic Jeremy's thinking was.

On Friday, all of us watched the storm grow even bigger. By Saturday, it was obvious that we were going to be hit and hit hard.

Katrina was a massive storm. The gaming commission finally made the call; casinos were to close at 2 a.m. on Sunday morning. Gerald and I discussed whether we should evacuate or stay. He was dealing with his medical issues and I was blind in one eye. What a pair we were!

When he and I left work on Saturday, we pretty much decided to stock up on water and non-perishable foods and just hunker down. We were tired of making the trek north and back in less than forty-eight hours. We'd just shelter in place.

At home, I had both the Weather Channel and my computer radar going. I watched the storm into the early morning hours. Somehow, I was able to sleep for a couple hours, then got up to monitor Katrina some more. It didn't look good.

Within a few minutes, it was clear we couldn't stay in our home. The authorities were calling for mandatory evacuations in many areas. Katrina's path was now three hundred miles wide. There was really no way to escape its wrath if we stayed put.

I woke Gerald and said, "We gotta go!"

He responded sleepily, "I thought we were going to ride it out."

I told him, "There's no way to ride this one out. It's huge and headed right for us. Probably a Category 4 or 5. Get up and get ready. I'm going to call the Horseshoe in Tunica to see if we can get a room." Finding accommodations would be tough. Most of the people we knew had already evacuated or else were stuck in miles of traffic, trying to get north to Tunica. But I crossed my fingers and gave it a try.

Calling the hotel itself didn't get any results. All of their rooms were gone. Finally, I was able to reach a friend I'd worked with up in Tunica. Miracle of miracles, he was able to get us accommodations. I knew the poker room had a block of rooms set aside and this is most likely how he managed to get us one. But however, he accomplished it, I was grateful.

Assuming we'd be back home in a day or two, Gerald and I grabbed some clean underwear, a couple of T-shirts and a couple of pairs of shorts. We didn't really think about protecting our house. After all, it was only eighteen months old.

We took back roads to avoid as much traffic as possible and get on our way. We'd danced this hurricane dance many times before so we knew the drill.

Between us, Gerald and I had about $100 in cash. He suggested we go to an ATM on the way out of Biloxi. I wasn't too concerned about money since we had our debit cards but because we were passing our bank branch, we stopped and got another few hundred dollars. Later, we were so glad we did because our bank was without power and there was no way to access cash.

It took us much longer than anticipated to make it to Tunica but we still managed to ditch a majority of the traffic jams. Gerald and I settled into our room and checked the weather on TV. We breathed a sigh of relief that we were out of Katrina's direct path. I felt like we could relax and try to have some fun.

It was like Homecoming Week because there were so many people we knew at the Horseshoe in Tunica, both dealers and players from the Gulf Coast. That Sunday evening there was a real party atmosphere. When we went to bed on August 28, we had no idea what we would wake up to.

•

Once again, as soon as I opened my eyes, I turned on the Weather Channel. It did not look good. There was no information coming out of Biloxi, which made me think Katrina hit pretty hard there. Everyone gathered in the poker room to share whatever they knew about the situation on the Coast. There was a lot of speculation but nothing specific.

The news still wasn't talking about Biloxi and what kind of damage it sustained. The levees in New Orleans had broken and the city was flooded. Understandably, the prime focus was on New Orleans and the horrible damage there, the hundreds of lives lost. We weren't able to get any reports about the Biloxi area until Tuesday morning. And it wasn't the news we'd hoped for.

They reported that a thirty-foot storm surge overran the city itself. For two full blocks, everything north of Biloxi Beach was washed away, including Gerald's and my doctor's offices. Our medical records were washed away with it. Beautiful antebellum homes across the road from the beach, structures that had withstood Hurricane Camille in 1969, were now vacant lots. What was the fate of our sweet, little homestead?

Gerald and I held onto the hope that because we weren't actually on the water, there was still a good chance that our house wasn't severely damaged. When I called Jeremy, he said that he'd get to Ocean Springs as soon as they allowed people in and would assess the damage.

Roads into Biloxi weren't cleared until Thursday, which is when Jeremy made his way to our house. I was expecting him to say, "The fence is down" or "Your palm plants were destroyed." But instead, he said, "Mom, you and Gerald don't need to come back here."

I was confused. "Why?" I asked. Jeremy took a deep breath and told me that EVERYTHING in the house was covered with mold because there'd been a foot of water in the house. Though the flood waters had receded, Jeremy could tell this by the watermark left on the walls. There was also a huge hole in the roof. Our house had to be gutted before it would be habitable.

I told Jeremy, "Save the important things, whatever's salvageable." He said he would.

After inspecting the house, Jeremy turned around and drove right back to Tuscaloosa. He picked up five of his crew members from the building project they'd been working on and took them to Biloxi where they completely gutted the house. They cut out the sheetrock and piled it on the lawn. Like all of our neighbors were going to have to do.

Unbelievably, Jeremy's crew completed the job in only a few hours. When he called to say they were done, I asked him to grab the clothes hanging in my closet. He said, "Mom, you don't understand. Everything is covered in black mold, from the wall on down. There's nothing worth saving."

Of course, Jeremy was right. Until that moment, it really hadn't registered that everything I owned and had saved over a lifetime was gone.

I was speechless.

Jeremy interrupted my thoughts. "Your sister wants you to call her," he said. "Aunt Berta's worried sick." I should have already checked in with her since I knew Alberta was probably glued to the TV, watching the Gulf Coast weather way up in Montana.

Throughout this difficult time, Jeremy was and continued to be my rock. I was so grateful to have him in my life.

When Berta answered the phone, she immediately said, "You guys need to come up here and figure out what you're going to do." I hesitated. "At least you'll have an address and a computer to better deal with what's to come," Berta pointed out. I thanked her and hung up.

Gerald shrugged when I asked what he thought about going to Montana. "Do we have any other offers?" he wondered. Typical Gerald.

Given our current circumstances, we decided Montana was our best bet for the time being. Gerald and I knew we were going to be out of a home and jobless for quite a while. The Grand Casino in Biloxi where we'd worked was actually blown out of the water and landed across the highway!

No home, no job, no question, we were going to Montana. I asked Berta to find a liver specialist for Gerald and an eye surgeon for me. My husband's autoimmune hepatitis required ongoing care and I was still blind in my right eye.

So, we gathered up our T-shirts and shorts and headed fifteen hundred miles north, diving headlong into the Montana fall and winter! YIKES!

But at least we had somewhere to go.

11

Baby, It's Cold Outside

On our way to Montana, it began to sink in that Gerald and I had lost nearly everything we owned. More than fifty years of memories and treasures are what devastated me the most. But losing all of that furniture, clothes and my massive collection of cooking equipment also hurt. I wiped a tear from my eye as I realized that Jeremy's baby book was gone too. I was the mom who filled out every page for every occasion. Pressed into that memory book was the little bracelet Jeremy wore in the hospital, a lock of his baby hair, and so much more. His first pair of shoes and childhood photographs were irreplaceable. All the rest was much less important.

My niece Shellie and her husband Dan suggested we stop at their place in Kansas on our way to Montana. She thought it was a good idea for us to stay there a couple of nights and gather our wits. Gerald and I agreed. My niece made arrangements with my two brothers, other sister and their families who live in the Kansas City area to meet, share a meal and talk about what had happened. We had a good visit, surrounded by love and support. Gerald and I were so moved that each of them brought something to contribute to our dire situation.

Later, we said our goodbyes to everyone and continued north.

When Gerald and I arrived in Montana on Saturday afternoon, my sister informed us that her neighbors had planned a pancake breakfast the next day at their community center in our honor. There, people gave both donations and goods to help meet our immediate needs. Again, Gerald and I were floored. What a welcoming community! We met some of the kindest, most generous people ever while we were holed up in Billings, Montana.

•

The fall brought pleasant weather to Big Sky Country. For us, winter unofficially began on October 30 with a bright, beautiful snowfall. While it was wonderful to look at, it was not so wonderful to navigate when you haven't driven in a snowy climate for many years.

That first snowstorm announced its presence with a power outage. We waited until it got pretty chilly in the house before deciding to get a hotel room that had heat and electricity. Welcome to Montana!

Of course, the cold and occasional snow persisted throughout the winter months. I was happy when spring came. Gerald and I had a date to go home to Mississippi as well as jobs to go home to. We were lucky. Many people had to permanently relocate and struggled for several years to find adequate work.

Berta and her husband Richard decided that they'd follow us home to the Gulf Coast and help transport some of the things we'd gathered while living in Montana. Gerald wasn't physically able to do a lot, so their help was immeasurable. I was surrounded by angels.

My sister and I became immersed in our "replacement mission." It was kind of fun to buy new furniture and fixtures but it was also bittersweet. We replaced the important, most necessary items and decided to keep things minimalistic. I realized that "stuff" means nothing. You can replace "stuff" in a few days. What I had to remember was to cherish the memories of the things that were destroyed, things that could never be replaced.

On August 29, 2006, the first anniversary of Hurricane Katrina, Gerald and I started our new jobs at the Beau Rivage. Most of the people we'd worked with before were there for orientation but we also saw some new faces. Everyone had their own unique survival stories and we were all very thankful to be back, to be alive.

Gerald and I rang in 2007 with gratitude that our friends had survived, that our home was rebuilt, that we had good jobs and that the entire Gulf Coast was on the mend.

But mostly, I was grateful for Jeremy and the role he played in our recovery. Without him, I don't know what we would have done.

12

Big Changes

In 2007, Jeremy's life was about to change dramatically. Nicely settled in Louisiana, he was in the middle of building a new apartment complex. Things were going well for him. Jeremy deserved every bit of his success because he was a hard worker and very skilled at what he did. He put his heart and soul into his career.

Early spring, Jeremy called and told me he was dating someone. He sounded very excited about this new woman, Jennifer, and I was very happy for him. Jeremy was never a "social animal," so he didn't date much. He had a great sense of humor, but he was also restrained. A lot of women didn't "get" him because he wasn't flashy or flamboyant.

As we talked, Jeremy mentioned that Jennifer had two very young children. One was less than a year old and the other was only two. It surprised me that Jeremy would get involved with a woman who had kids because when he was younger, Jeremy had said he didn't think he'd have children. The idea of having no grandbabies made my spirit sink but I was totally supportive if that was his decision.

I explained to Jeremy that at thirty-two, it was likely that any woman about the same age would have at least one child. So, he should consider it carefully before getting serious about the relationship with Jennifer. He promised me that he would.

In September of that year, Jeremy phoned to say that he'd asked Jennifer to marry him. He loved her and was more than willing to take on the responsibility of both a wife and her children. In November 2007, Jennifer, Jeremy and her kids Will and Emma moved in together.

Since my job required me to work weekends and Jeremy was working six or seven days a week on his building projects, it was difficult to get together, especially since we lived 250 miles apart. This and the fact that Gerald's medical problems worsened made it even harder to meet. But we had faith that we'd be able to get together soon.

•

Besides having autoimmune hepatitis, Gerald was diagnosed with a condition called ascites, directly caused by his hepatitis. The ascites made his abdomen swell from fluid buildup. Because of it, Gerald could no longer work and eventually had to go to the hospital every week to have the excess fluid drained from his belly. But through it all, my sweet husband kept his easy-going personality.

Despite these obstacles, I hoped we'd be able to plan holiday time with Jeremy—and that we'd finally get to meet Jennifer and her children. But a couple of weeks before Thanksgiving, all plans were put on hold when Gerald lost his balance and fell, scraping his arm badly on our textured wall. Because he was also diabetic, we were very concerned that Gerald's wound wouldn't heal properly since infection is a big danger to diabetics.

At the same time, Gerald complained of shoulder pain. While the scrape healed nicely, his shoulder wasn't getting better. A couple of weeks before Christmas, Gerald decided to go for an x-ray. I'll never forget, it was a Friday, I was cleaning house and suggested he run up to the doctor's office and then to the hospital for the x-ray. Both were less than a mile from our home. By the time Gerald came back, I'd be finished cleaning and we could go to the casino and play poker. A busman's holiday, but I guess poker was our job as well as our recreation.

Gerald wasn't gone very long. He'd had the x-ray after visiting the doctor and came home. Before we could leave for the casino, the doctor's office called. They asked him to go back to the hospital to redo the x-ray. At first, we didn't think much of it. We figured the image was blurred and they needed a better picture. So, Gerald went back to the hospital and I waited at home.

I began to get concerned when he didn't come back for quite some time. One hour, two hours passed. I was getting anxious. When Gerard finally called, the news wasn't good. "You need to come to the hospital," he said, his voice shaky. "They say I either have tuberculosis or I have cancer!"

How could this be possible? My husband went in for a simple shoulder x-ray! Now he was telling me that he could have a life-threatening disease. I assured Gerald, "I'll be right there" and was out of the house in two minutes and at the hospital in five.

Once in the emergency room, they took me to the examination room where Gerald was waiting. His face was as white as the hospital gown he was wearing.

Stunned, I asked what was going on. Gerald explained that the x-ray showed a problem with his lungs. I knew it couldn't be TB because he had no symptoms. As far as lung damage, Gerald never smoked and had never had a breathing problem. I thought they must have made a mistake. But sadly, they hadn't.

The medical team was trying to decide whether or not to admit Gerald. Eventually, they did check him into the hospital and ran a barrage of tests. The next day, they told us that Gerald had lung cancer but the lab work showed it hadn't spread. We were so relieved. They discussed treatment and mentioned fixing his rotator cuff, the original injury he was in to have x-rayed. At least we had a plan! But not for long.

The next morning, everything changed. Gerald's doctor came in with extremely bad news. They sent the biopsy to another laboratory and the results came back quite differently—it confirmed that Gerald did, in fact, have lung cancer that had probably spread.

After lots of tests and tears, they discovered that Gerald also had liver cancer. It seemed the cancer had actually started in his liver and metastasized to his lungs. Probably to other parts of his body as well. They'd know for sure in a few days.

My sweet, kind, loving Gerald was dying!

I left his room and stumbled to the parking lot, trembling like a leaf. I needed something to calm my nerves but couldn't figure out what. Glancing up, I noticed a convenience store across the street from the hospital. Without even thinking, I went and bought a pack of cigarettes. Keep in mind, I'd quit nine months earlier. A devoted smoker for forty years, I stopped cold turkey for Gerald's health. But now his health was shot to hell so what difference did it make?

I lit up, took a deep drag and went back to my car. Then I called Jeremy, my rock, my foundation. "Gerald has terminal cancer," I gasped.

My son was in the middle of an important construction job in Louisiana. All he said was, "Where are you?"

I told him.

"I'm on my way," Jeremy said.

I was still sitting in that hospital parking lot when Jeremy drove up three hours later. I got out of my car, cigarette in hand. Jeremy just looked at me, his soulful eyes filled with pity. He didn't say a word. All he did was hug me. I let the tears and fears go, and for a brief moment, felt like I was okay. But just for a minute.

13

Saying Goodbye

The first week of January 2008, I called my sister Berta and asked if she and Richard could come to Mississippi to help with Gerald. I needed to work as much as possible to support us and by then, Gerald needed someone at home with him. He was on oxygen, sleeping a lot and not eating much.

Although I never told Gerald, at the time of his diagnosis, I'd asked the doctor how long he thought Gerald had left. The doctor looked at me sadly and said, "Maybe two months." I asked him not to tell Gerald unless he asked. He never did.

Berta and Richard arrived as soon as they could. Because of the Family Medical Leave Act (FMLA), I was able to work on the nights Gerald wasn't feeling well and use my leave days to spend with him when he was doing better. The system worked out for us and Gerald had constant care thanks to Berta and Richard pitching in.

Jeremy came to visit for Mardi Gras, which was early February that year. Gerald was feeling pretty good that day and really wanted to go to the casino for their Mardi Gras festivities. They usually made a big deal about Mardi Gras with costumes, little parades, music and such. I knew Gerald was running out of time so I wanted him to be able to see his friends at the casino, and hopefully, be strong enough to play poker.

We loaded the wheelchair I'd rented from a medical supply store into the car and headed to the casino. Gerald was so glad to see his friends and former coworkers. He even attempted to play poker. But by that time, Gerald's cancer had most likely begun to attack his brain. He couldn't complete simple tasks and had trouble concentrating on the cards in his hands. He tried to brush it off as no big deal but I knew it bothered him.

Everyone was happy to see Gerald. He had a great time and even wanted to stop for pizza on the way home. This would be the last time Gerald left the house.

•

On Valentine's Day, Berta and Richard said they needed to go home for a week or so to take care of some personal business. They promised to return as soon as they could. I decided to stay home from work and enjoy whatever time Gerald and I had left. Neither of us spoke about him dying. Like the five-hundred-pound elephant in the room, we ignored it.

That Valentine's night, Gerald started to have trouble breathing. No matter what we tried, he couldn't get comfortable. We moved him from the bed to the couch to the floor and back again. I told him, "Tomorrow, I'm going to get you a hospital bed if I have to go to the hospital and roll one down the road myself." Gerald gave a small laugh. Because the funny thing was, he knew I would have tried it.

The next morning, I contacted a hospice service to see what they could provide in the way of support. They told me that if Gerald's doctor verified that he'd be having no further treatment, the hospice team would bring everything my husband needed to be comfortable. Including a hospital bed.

At 2 p.m. that very same afternoon, hospice arrived like a SWAT team. A nurse, a counselor and an intake person sat with us to assess Gerald's condition. After evaluating him, they told me as kindly as possible that he probably only had a few days left. This was all so hard for me to comprehend. Only a few days ago, Gerald was up and about, and at least could enjoy watching television. A few weeks earlier, he was at the casino, laughing with friends, and enjoying a slice of pizza afterwards. Now his days were numbered, literally. How could this be?

I gathered what strength I could muster and watched the hospice workers transfer Gerald to the hospital bed they'd brought. Palliative care had begun.

I called Berta and told her that Gerald might not make it much longer. She and Richard immediately booked a flight to return to Mississippi. Although Gerald wasn't close to his siblings, I contacted them. I explained to his sister and two brothers that if they wanted to see Gerald again, they would need to get here within forty-eight hours.

Next, I called Jeremy. "I'm on my way," he said once again. He and Gerald had become very close over the past few years. I believe my son held a special place in his heart for the man who made his mother so happy.

The next day was Saturday. I had no idea that night would be the last Gerald and I would spend alone together. On Sunday, my sister and brother-in-law arrived. Late in the afternoon on Monday, Gerald's siblings came. We had a full house.

That Monday evening, the hospice nurse and aide were in Gerald's room bathing him and monitoring him. I heard someone call, "The nurse says you need to come in…it's time."

I went into the room with my sister, climbed up into the hospital bed with Gerald and held him while Berta sang the hymn "Be Not Afraid" to my husband and held his hand. In just a few moments, Gerald drew his last breath in my arms.

On February 18, 2008, the sweetest, kindest man I'd ever known was dead at fifty-four.

14

Alone Again

Just eighteen months after beginning our recovery from the from the wrath of Hurricane Katrina, I found myself alone again. Somehow, I had to muster the strength to return to work and once more, start over. Thanks to good friends, I had a strong support system. And Jeremy was my rock through everything.

For two whole years, from the spring of 2008 until the spring of 2010, I carried on working and doing little else. I was like a robot on autopilot. Every couple of months, I'd take an extra day off and drive to Jeremy's for a weekend visit. It was great getting to spoil Jennifer's kids, who were just darling. Because Jeremy was so busy with his career, I felt lucky to spend time with him whenever I could. It meant so much to me and kept me going.

•

When spring came, the planning and preparation for Jeremy and Jennifer's wedding was in full swing. Originally, they weren't going to have a big shindig but I felt that as my only child, I wanted Jeremy's wedding to be special. (Okay, maybe a little bit for me too.) After all, he was thirty-five and had every intention of this being his only marriage.

As my gift to them, I offered pay for the wedding ceremony and reception—as long as Jeremy and Jennifer planned it. They were moved and told me that my offer was extremely generous, and to my delight, accepted. I have to say, they put together a beautiful, intimate celebration of their love.

In June 2010, Jeremy's family and friends came from Missouri, Kansas, Tennessee and Montana to share in his special day. Jennifer had a few friends and family there as well. It was an outdoor, evening wedding and the Mississippi weather did not disappoint. The temperature was 105 degrees. Somehow, Jennifer managed to be an hour late for her own wedding! The guests were getting restless—and hot.

When the bride finally made her appearance, the wedding went off without a hitch. Her relatives had prepared a *cochon de lait,* a Cajun whole roasted, suckling pig. They sure set out a delicious spread of food. The festivities included the usual wedding traditions, like the mother/son dance. During it, my niece Shellie sang "The Man You've Become." It's a poignant song about a son will always be his momma's boy, no matter how old he is. It fit Jeremy and me to a T. Of course, I cried. Many others did too.

•

One Friday night in March the following year, I was feeling ill. I remember vomiting for over an hour. I'd never experienced anything like this before and I was worried. I called a friend and asked him to take me to the emergency room. By the time we drove the short distance to the hospital, I had become alarmingly short of breath. That's when I knew this was something pretty serious. Maybe I was having a heart attack.

In the ER, they immediately put me in a trauma bay as the medical team tried to assess what was wrong with me. A nurse drew blood to run tests. The results came back negative for any cardiac incident. I got more concerned at that report because now I *really* had no idea what it could be. Was I dying? I got horrible flashbacks of Gerald, going to get an x-ray and finding out he had terminal cancer.

My friend stuck his head in the door and said, "I've called Jeremy and he's on his way from Louisiana." I knew it would be hours before he arrived, so I told my friend, "If I don't make it, tell Jeremy I love him with all my heart."

I don't recall everything that happened after that but I was admitted to a room and given something to help me sleep.

The following day, the cardiologist told me they wanted to perform an angiogram. This test scared the pants off me because in it, they thread a catheter into your groin area and up through the blood vessels in your heart to check for any kind of blockage.

Although I was afraid of the angiogram procedure, it was the only way they could find out what was wrong with me. I was young. I had too much to live for—Jeremy and Jennifer and my new step-grandkids. Reluctantly, I agreed to the angiogram.

All I remember is them wheeling me into the operating room. The next thing I remember is waking up on the gurney in the hallway with Jeremy and a doctor standing over me. The doctor said, "We need to schedule you for open-heart surgery tomorrow. You have a severe blockage in several places."

My response to him was, "Not tomorrow. Tomorrow is my birthday!"

The doctor agreed to do the surgery the day after my birthday. So, I spent my sixty-second birthday in a hospital bed watching a video of an open-heart surgery. Everyone thought I was crazy for doing that but I wanted to know what was going to happen to me!

Let's just say that the next four or five days were not something I'd like to repeat. The first two were the roughest. Jeremy was staying at my house while I recovered. He spent time with me at the hospital, bringing me things to eat and drink that he probably shouldn't have. Jeremy stayed in Mississippi until I was back home and arranged to have someone look in on me. My son thought of everything and was such a caring man. *I must have done something right,* I thought.

•

Unfortunately, 2012 brought another surgery. I had a repetitive-motion injury to my shoulder due to dealing cards for over a decade. It couldn't be ignored anymore. I was in constant pain; my range of motion was affected and my shoulder had to be fixed.

Now I was in a pickle! After my shoulder surgery, I'd need help with almost everything since my arm would be in a sling for several weeks. Because of the nature of his work, it wasn't practical for Jeremy to come stay with me. So he arrived with his truck, loaded up my portable bed and everything else I would need and took me home with him after I had the operation.

I stayed with Jeremy and his family for about ten days. It was great to spend time with them, even under those circumstances. I was used to living alone and truth be told, sometimes it was lonely. Being in a house with two active kids was a welcome change.

Jeremy had always been my lifeline. We started discussing my retirement, which was only a couple of years away. He suggested that I sell my house and come live with them. Since he was a little boy, Jeremy had always said, "When you get too old to work, Mama, I will always take care of you." And he meant it.

His wife Jennifer was onboard 100%. She explained that when Jeremy proposed to her, he said, "You need to know that if you marry me, my mom comes with the deal. I'm always going to look after her." It felt good to be wanted, to be cared for, especially after being on my own since Gerald died.

Wasting no time, Jeremy started designing and planning for building a new home with a mother's apartment. For me.

15

Spring Fling

By the spring of 2013, things appeared to be going well for both Jeremy's family and me. I was already counting the months until my retirement. Jeremy was working on a large commercial shopping center project and was putting in a lot of hours, plus weekends.

But suddenly, whenever I talked to Jeremy, I noticed that he sounded "down." Although my son was never a gregarious person, I knew him well enough to read even the smallest inflections in his voice. He seemed tired, withdrawn. We talked about the impact the demands of his job were having on his family time but he assured me that the project was going well and that he was just beat. With a wife and two small children to support, combined with a stressful work situation, that sounded reasonable to me.

However, a couple of weeks later, when Jeremy called me one evening, I knew something was up—he rarely called at night. The first thing he said was, "Mom, Jennifer's cheating on me!" I was shocked and crushed but tried to hide it.

Immediately, I asked if his wife's lover was the guy who'd been her best friend for many years. "No," he said. I was even more surprised when he told me, "It's her best girlfriend!"

Now, that's the last thing I expected to hear. I asked Jeremy if he was sure and he assured me that he was. He'd suspected something might be going on so he put a camera in their bedroom. That camera captured several different incidents of the affair. I was silent for a minute, then asked, "What are you going to do?"

Jeremy shot back, "I'm getting a divorce." Then he continued, "Mom, I told her before we got married that there were only two things in the world that would ever make me leave: lying and cheating. And I meant it." He hesitated. "I can never trust her again and I don't want that kind of constant question in my marriage."

I reminded Jeremy that Jennifer might cut him off from the kids and he had no legal claim to them since he hadn't adopted them. Jeremy choked up a little and admitted, "I know but I'm going to do everything I can to stay civil with her so that doesn't happen." Jeremy was the only dad they knew and Jennifer realized that Jeremy was not only good *for* them but he was good *to* them.

Besides that, from the time she met Jeremy, Jennifer never had to work one day outside the home. He wanted her to be able to devote all of her time and attention to the kids. Jeremy didn't even make an issue about the fact that their biological father didn't pay any child support. Unlike their biological dad, Jeremy was deeply committed to those children.

It hit me hard when I realized that my relationship with my step grandkids Will and Emma was going to change a great deal. I know I was never my daughter-in-law's favorite person in the world (and whose mother-in-law is?) but we were always civil to each other. Now Jennifer would owe me nothing. Not respect, not even the right to see her kids. I feared that my grandchildren would disappear from my life before they ever really got to know me. But I hoped for the best.

•

Jeremy moved all of his belongings from their house and bunked with two good friends who happened to be co-workers. By the time the divorce was finalized, it was almost the end of the year. Somehow, he'd managed to maintain his relationship with the kids—unless and until Jennifer got mad at him. I felt better knowing her children were still a part of our lives, at least for the time being.

I knew all of this was going to affect our plans of having a home together. Or at the very least, one I could afford when I retired. But I also knew that Jeremy had enough on his plate as it was so I gave him time to come to grips with his life change before I brought my situation up for discussion.

But retirement was looming on the horizon. I was eligible to stop working that March, when I'd turn sixty-five. Although I'd start getting Social Security and Medicare, it wouldn't be enough income for me to remain in my current home. Singlehandedly carrying a mortgage and covering my other expenses would be difficult, if not impossible. And after my shoulder surgery, I wasn't going to be able to continue working for long.

When Jeremy and I discussed the situation, we agreed that the best solution for all our problems would be for him and I to find a place near his work in Louisiana. We settled on an April move in date.

In the meantime, Jeremy and I planned to update my home in Mississippi and put it on the market. 2014 was a bad time to be selling a house but we had no choice, it had to be done.

Jeremy searched for suitable housing that gave each of us privacy while, at the same time, accommodated our needs. With all of his construction tools and equipment, the place would also have to come with some type of garage storage.

After a bit of legwork, Jeremy found a three bedroom, two bath single family home with an attached garage. He signed a lease that began on April 8.

Everything was falling into place nicely but it gave us little time to update my house and put it on the market. Until I sold it, I'd have to make mortgage payments on it plus pay half the rent on the new place. But with the help of Jeremy's friend Chuck and my friend Mary, we were able to get the house on the market by the first of May.

As quickly as I could, I packed up my house for our April 8 move. Jeremy made sure to be there when the guys loaded the truck. Then he and I headed to the new house, which was a two-and-a-half-hour drive away. The moving crew unpacked the truck and I began putting the house in order.

It was a good fit. Jeremy had the master suite and I had a TV/office room as well as my own bedroom and bath. Our private spaces were on opposite ends of the house, which was perfect for privacy, but we shared common areas like the kitchen, living and dining rooms.

Although Jeremy and I had a lot of personality traits in common, the biggest difference was that I had no patience and he was a procrastinator. As soon as something was possible, I wanted to work out all the details and get the job done. He, on the other hand, put off tasks way past the last possible moment.

So, in just a day or two, I had the house all set up, everything unpacked and in place. Jeremy still had a few unpacked boxes in his closet when we moved three years later.

Jeremy also liked to keep "stuff." After I lost everything in Hurricane Katrina, I decided that I was going to live with the minimal number of possessions. I had lost it all once so this time around, I only wanted to keep things that were useful and had sentimental value. In three months' time, Jeremy had filled the garage to the point that my car would never see the inside of it. Granted, most of his it was work equipment but there was a whole lot of useless stuff as well.

My old house was on the market. Jeremy and I we were established in our new place and all was well with our world. For now.

16

Escape Hatch

Before I retired, a woman who played poker at the casino where I worked in Mississippi learned I was moving to Louisiana. She suggested I might want to investigate starting a private poker game in the area. Several existed but she felt that the neighborhood where she lived had the potential to host another game. I told her I'd give it some thought.

Private poker games are legal if you don't take what's called a "rake." Essentially, a rake is where the host of the game skims a certain percentage of each pot to offset the cost of facilitating the game. The "income" from private games is solely from the players tipping the dealer. The "tip" generally equals what the rake would be. The legal difference is that charging a rake for players to play makes it a business which required a license. By only accepting tips, the players are voluntarily giving you a gratuity, which is totally legal.

Jeremy and I discussed the idea and decided that a private poker room could be a good source of supplemental income in my retirement. We found a small building that had been a restaurant in a former life and did a bit of remodeling. Next, we bought all the poker paraphernalia: tables, chairs, chips and a safe to protect our earnings. We were all set.

At first, he and I decided to host games just two days a week—Thursday and Sunday—and began to spread the word. Because I'd been a professional poker dealer for twenty years, people trusted that I knew how to run a professional game. And that I did. Jeremy was with me whenever we were open, not only to learn how to deal (and give me bathroom breaks) but to ensure my safety.

It was an all-cash business and I didn't leave the building without Jeremy and the protection he provided. It worked out well. We ended up keeping the private games going for about a year. We made some money, and best of all, it gave me the excuse to spend some quality time with my son.

•

Jeremy always had a good relationship with his dad David. As a youngster, Jeremy spent a few summers with him but he didn't really care for David's wife. So, he tried not to hang out with them as a couple, if he could help it.

As Jeremy got older, he and David both developed a keen interest in gold mining. Jeremy watched all the mining shows on television and researched the hobby, like he did everything that piqued his curiosity. As a result, Jeremy and David started to take mining trips to places like Colorado, Arizona and California. They'd spend two weeks on their adventures and come home with little jars with tiny gold flakes in them. But the best part was the father/son bonding.

In May 2015, Jeremy and his dad took their last mining trip together. David had been sick with hepatitis and liver disease for a few years. When Jeremy returned from that trip, he told me that he noticed his dad was getting sicker.

For some reason, instead of flying there, David had driven to Arizona. On his return trip to Missouri, David felt more and more ill. As soon as he arrived home, David ended up in the hospital. Not long after, Jeremy received a phone call from David's wife, saying they'd moved his dad to hospice. They didn't expect him to live much longer. Jeremy immediately booked a flight to Kansas City and went to his father's side. Two days later, David passed away at the age of sixty-four.

•

Around the summer of 2015, our poker game endeavor was winding down. It wasn't anything Jeremy or I had done wrong; it was just due to the fact that people taking breaks from gambling or focused on other commitments. Oh, well. It was fun while it lasted.

Soon after we closed its doors, Jeanne and Dominic, our lifelong friends from Kansas City and part of the origival tribe, stopped by to visit for a couple of days. They had just finished vacationing with their grandsons in Nashville and excitedly told me all the details about taking the kids to something called an escape room. I apologized, stopped them and called Jeremy in. "You need to listen to this," I told him.

I urged Jeanne and Dominic to explain the whole concept to Jeremy. They said that an escape room was a type of game where you were "trapped" in a themed room (or rooms). Participants were faced with the challenge of finding their way out of that place. Planted in the room were a series of clues. You had to solve a puzzle of sorts in order to advance in the game. If you found all the clues, you got out of escape the room.

I thought building our very own escape room would be a great business opportunity for Jeremy and me. There was nothing like it in the area. With Jeremy's construction expertise and creativity, I knew that he could create something like that with no problem.

After Jeanne and Dominic left, Jeremy and I sat down for a serious discussion about opening an escape room. We picked four themes Jeremy believed he could easily build rooms for. Next, he started working on puzzles, clues and researching existing escape rooms.

Today, there are thousands of escape rooms across the country and all over the world but there were only about three hundred in the United States back in 2015. We decided that Jeremy should make a trip to Florida to visit escape rooms there. Meanwhile, I would investigate everything on the business end, starting with estimates of what the startup would cost.

Thankfully, we'd saved most of the money we made from the private poker game and in February, my house sold, so we had a few thousand dollars to work with. Although it didn't sound like enough to start up a business, I forged ahead to compile the most realistic estimated cost I could.

I was well aware that only a small percentage of startup businesses make it past the first year and I sure didn't want to waste what little money we had. But I researched the heck out of this thing and was confident we could make a go of it.

Even though Jeremy was the ultimate procrastinator, he was excited about the possibilities of starting our escape room and immediately dove into it. He worked double-time figuring out possible themes, clues and mysteries to solve. He also scouted out possible locations, all this while working full time in construction.

I must admit, I thought I already knew all of my son's strengths but I was totally floored by the depth of his creativity. He figured out all the rooms, how to build them out and how the clues would mesh and flow together so participants could complete the games. I was able to add a few finishing touches but Jeremy was the true creative genius while I was the pragmatic businesswoman. We were a team that worked well together.

After finding a space to lease and putting together a solid business plan, Jeremy and I were ready to take the plunge. During our research, we knew that almost no one in our area had heard of escape rooms. The only family entertainment in town was the go-cart place, bowling alleys and movies. Since we had a very limited marketing budget (read that as almost nothing), we knew we would live or die by word-of-mouth advertising.

The next step was to have a very simple but eye-catching website built where tickets could be purchased. The website highlighted how the Escape Room offered a great opportunity for team-building exercises and was also an innovative place to hold birthday celebrations. It emphasized that we had four different themed rooms and encouraged folks to try them all. The website looked great but would people bite?

•

Nervous and excited, Jeremy and I set the Escape Room's grand opening for January 15, 2016. Honestly, we were terrified! We didn't want to be embarrassed by having no customers but knew that it was a real possibility no one would come. Our business plan set aside three months' worth of overhead in case we had no income during those initial months. Besides that cushion, there was no escape hatch. It was do or die.

Jeremy and I worked long days and into the night but come January 15, we opened the doors of the Escape Room, as scheduled. From that Friday on, we started making money. Truly, we were amazed at the response we got. Everyone loved it. Very quickly, we went from having two employees to five.

In April, not three months later, Jeremy came to me and said, "We need to lease the other half of this building."

My initial response was, "Are you crazy? We just got these four rooms up and running."

"We're doing well," Jeremy assured me. "But I know we can do even better." He swore that in six months, he could have four more rooms done in the other half of the building. The business would continue to grow, he was sure of it.

I couldn't help but agree with Jeremy's dreams of expansion. As it was, we were not only selling out but we were selling a unique experience. Once people completed all four of our escape rooms, they were itching for more. And by creating more escape rooms, we could offer them more.

But our pending expansion would be too much for Jeremy to manage while still working his construction business full time. We decided that in May, he would give up his construction career and devote all his efforts toward the Escape Room. When we were done building the new place, he could always pick construction back up again if he wanted to.

Since Jeremy would be busy getting the new rooms up and running as well as maintaining the existing games, this made perfect sense. We were profitable and the business could afford to pay him a salary. I wasn't taking any money out of the profits since I was able to live on my Social Security.

As business manager, I made sure everything was budgeted and that Jeremy didn't get carried away. But that didn't last long. As the project progressed, Jeremy came up with all sorts of cool things to add to the escape rooms. These new games contained lots of electronic components. We also decided to add a "party room" on that side that could host kids' birthday parties since these quickly became some of our greatest sources of revenue.

By fall, Jeremy and I realized that the only Halloween entertainment in our area was a pretty lame "haunted trail." Basically, you walked outside in the woods and scary stuff popped out at you or was placed among the trees. Fun until you do it. Then it's one and done. Jeremy knew there was a market for a Halloween-themed escape room, so he built one.

Again, my son's instincts were right. Jeremy's creepy "serial killer" room sold out each and every night.

17

Derailed

Things were great between Jeremy and me. We worked together well and we lived with each other well. We respected each other's privacy and gave each other personal space. My life goal at that point was to do everything I could to help make Jeremy successful at whatever he chose to do. He always worked hard, always tried to be good and kind to other people—and he succeeded. I wanted him to enjoy his life and the time he had with his step kids as much as he could. He was very involved with every aspect of their lives.

But all of that was to change very soon.

•

The fall of 2016 marked the beginning of the train going off the rails for me. As Jeremy worked on the Halloween escape room, I noticed that he was spending less and less time at the business and when he was there, he often disappeared for an hour or more. It seemed like I was always looking for him: calling his cell phone with no response, texting him, leaving voice mails for him.

I soon discovered that Jeremy was hanging out a lot with a young woman. Richelle was a waitress at a Mexican restaurant he frequented. She was nearly twenty years his junior. I started hearing all sorts of things from my employees about this girl Richelle and they weren't very flattering. Before long, I was sure she was a negative distraction in his life. I had no choice but to confront Jeremy about it. He and I were always able to have rational conversations about anything so I thought this talk would be the same.

One day, I sat down with Jeremy and told him flat out that I felt he was neglecting the Escape Room. I wondered what in the world he was doing that worth jeopardizing our new endeavor. Business was thriving, bringing in a half million dollars in the first year. We were debt-free and able to support ourselves as well as several employees.

Of course, Jeremy didn't see it quite the same way. He felt he was doing everything he needed to sustain and grow the business. I took a deep breath and ventured into discussing Richelle. According to what I'd heard, she had more negatives than positives, the biggest of which was a "past" drug problem.

Point blank, I asked Jeremy what Richelle brought to the table. She was twenty-two, had a child she'd lost custody of due to drug use, a dead-end job, no money, no life experience. In short, she had nothing Jeremy should hitch his star to, especially considering his lifestyle and successes. As far as I knew, Jeremy was never a drinker nor did he do drugs. He didn't even smoke marijuana. My son was a straight arrow. All of his friends confirmed this.

Jeremy's response was pretty much, "We have a lot of common interests like music and we have good conversations." That was it.

I literally ended up begging Jeremy to turn his attentions toward people who were at the same stage in their lives as he was. Or at least closer to his age. He was forty-one and Richelle was almost half his age. I mean, how mature were YOU at twenty-two? I know I was a real wild child.

My best efforts to steer Jeremy away from Richelle didn't work. I pleaded with him, reminding him that he knew I'd never give him advice that wasn't in his best interest. Everything I ever told him was what I truly believed was the right thing for him. Although Jeremy agreed that I always had his best interest in mind, he still refused to stop seeing Richelle. He said they would always be friends. I had a bad feeling in the pit of my gut about this Richelle woman but tried to let it go.

•

For the remainder of 2016, I tried my best to comprehend why Jeremy was behaving this way. What power did this woman have over him? Was it sex? Was he lonely? What need did Richelle fill that his work, his kids, his friends and his mom didn't fill?

Jeremy continued to dodge work, stay away from home more frequently and gradually, began spending more and more money. Although he was getting paid very well from the Escape Room, he was always asking for more money with one excuse or another. Sometimes, he even took cash out of the business account without my knowing until I'd reconciled the bank account. When I questioned him about these mysterious withdrawals, he'd come up with some sort of flimsy excuse.

Jeremy and I decided to move when it came time to renew the lease on our rental home—our rent had increased yet again. We had our sights set on a four-bedroom place so each of the kids had their own bedroom when they stayed overnight. They were getting older and needed their privacy. Our new digs also needed a big garage or workshop to house Jeremy's construction tools and his ever-growing collection of rocks and mining finds.

We were fortunate to find the perfect place less than a half mile from where we were currently living. The four-bedroom house was laid out so that the master bedroom suite and the other bedrooms were separated by the kitchen and living room. This made it more like a "roommate" set up with the personal spaces at either end of the house. It also had a great, big deck off of the dining area. The house sat on three acres, which included a shop *and* a barn. There was plenty of room for whatever we needed.

Jeremy and I both fell in love with the house and planned to move in on April Fool's Day. It was already the middle of March, so we wasted no time. We quickly set up an appointment to meet at the leasing office, sign paperwork, pay the deposit and the first month's rent. The financial aspect wasn't a problem since I had at least $5,000 put away in the safe in Jeremy's room. This is where he stored his guns and where we kept our cash. We'd been doing it for years. Having a safe was a "must" when we were doing the private poker room and we'd had a safe ever since.

When we arrived at the leasing office, Jeremy had the bank bag tucked under his arm with all the necessary cash in it. After the rental agent gave us the total amount we owed, Jeremy opened the bag and had this strange look on his face. "Oh damn," he said. "I must have grabbed the wrong bag." Even though we had two or three bank bags in the safe, I still thought this was strange. I tried to shrug it off as I wrote a check. We finished up and started home.

Jeremy was fidgety on the car ride home but I credited it to him knowing that he'd made a dumb mistake by not checking the bag. Everyone messes up once in a while. But it turned out fine, the papers were signed and we'd soon be in our new place.

Back at the house, Jeremy's story about the missing money changed. Now he claimed that when he'd gone on a fishing trip with his friend Harvey to the Gulf Coast, he had about $4,000 in his pants pocket. The last time he saw the money was when he pulled it out to give a tip to the fishing guide. But now that wad of cash was gone. It must have fallen out of his pants, he said.

That fish tale was just too far-fetched for me to be believe. I told Jeremy that if he was that careless with money, things would have to change. Especially since he'd been overspending. I was going to take charge of *all* the finances, his personal bills and the company money. Jeremy would get a set amount of cash each week and have to learn to live within those means. Jeremy's only personal costs were his gas, cigarettes and a few other miscellaneous expenses. I would handle everything else related to the business and our living expenses.

I took Jeremy's checkbook, personal debit card, the company debit card and checks. He really didn't put up much of a fight because he knew I was dead serious. No argument or fish tale he devised could hold up against cold, hard reality.

And no, I didn't think I was treating him like a child. True, Jeremy was a grown man in his forties but our business partnership and his financial future were on the table. Besides, in addition to being his business partner, I was also his mother, with his best interest top of mind. Jeremy and I agreed that he would receive a generous "allowance" of $500 a week.

Although I didn't want to make him feel like a high school kid, I thought that amount was far more than Jeremy needed. I even suggested that he not carry it all with him and maybe, just maybe, at the end of the week, he might find that he even had money left over. But unfortunately, it didn't quite work out that way.

Jeremy was fine for a few weeks but then, by Wednesday or Thursday, he started asking for more money. When I questioned what he was spending it on, he really couldn't give me a reasonable answer. This worried me. But I knew he only had access to the funds I was giving him so occasionally, I'd slip him the extra $100 he asked for. But I was baffled as to where all that money was going. And he wasn't telling.

It didn't take me long to figure out that something was going on, something so bad that Jeremy didn't want me to know. I talked myself into believing that he was spending the money on Richelle. Supporting her, buying her jewelry and her fancy clothes. That's the only thing that made any sense to me. Because I knew Jeremy had been more than generous with other girlfriends, it seemed to be the logical conclusion. Although I was not happy about it one bit, I thought he'd have to stop showering Richelle with his money when it ran out.

I had no idea what was in store for us.

18

Bombshell

Things carried on pretty much the same and I was at a loss at what to do.

How do you parent a forty-two-year-old? I knew how to be Jeremy's mother, his friend and his business partner but I was confused as to what my role as a parent should be. To me, the word "parent" is a verb. It's active, it's kinetic. But parenting an adult is different. It evolves, it changes as they grow. It's hard to know when to pull back and when to push harder.

Plus, it's difficult to get a grown-ass man in his forties to do what you want him to do, even if it's to his benefit. You can't make demands. You can only ask and eventually beg, which is what I did. It was pathetic but I knew Jeremy was on a crash course to a bad place. Although I didn't know the details of what he was into, I knew it wasn't good.

Jeremy and I always had well-defined boundaries, even as housemates. But after I was forced to take over all the finances, the paradigm shifted. I found myself watching everything he was doing with a critical eye. I second-guessed the information he shared. Since he was staying away from home and the business often, again, I thought it had to do with Richelle, this trashy girl he was so enamored with. It was so difficult for me to believe that Jeremy lived a life of lies and deceit when we had been closer than any mother and son I knew.

Before 2016, I would have fought anyone tooth and nail who even suggested that Jeremy was lying to me. He had never been in any trouble anywhere. Not in school, not at work, not with the police. The only encounter he ever had with law enforcement was a speeding ticket. So, it was very hard for me to doubt my son.

But being inquisitive by nature, I drove myself to the point of watching every move he made. By the end of 2017, I was questioning myself and everything that was going on. Was I imagining it? Was I making more of it than I should have been?

But one thing was clear, I had doubts about my son that I never thought I would have. What was Jeremy doing that was so awful that he was hiding it from me?

•

2018 started out much the same: Jeremy making himself scarce and me wondering why? It didn't seem logical that he would be tangled up with Richelle for so long without trying to help me understand their relationship. How serious was it?

I knew he'd never marry her but I couldn't fathom why he was spending so much time with this woman.

I'd had convinced myself that by now, Jeremy was definitely supporting Richelle. I didn't know to what extent but there was no other explanation for the money Jeremy was spending that he refused to account for. He knew that supporting Richelle was something I would disapprove of so he kept it from me. At least that's what I tried to convince myself.

When February rolled around, Jeremy started not coming home more frequently. What previously had been the occasional night of staying out became every single night. When I asked when he was coming home, Jeremy's answer was always, "In a couple of days" or "On the weekend." But days, weekends passed, and no Jeremy.

•

Finally, by the end of February, I decided to take a stand. Jeremy was behaving so out of character that no matter how I tried to reason it out in my head, I couldn't grasp why he was avoiding coming home and continuing to lie about it. Enough was enough.

I texted Jeremy a very long message—because I wanted it all in writing. In the text, I explained that I needed to know what his plans were. I told him that I didn't move to Louisiana and work so hard to help him succeed in his own business, only for him to desert our home and our business. I also told him that if he planned to keep living somewhere else, I would be forced to get a smaller house, plus reevaluate our business agreement. Jeremy was benefiting from all the business profits and wasn't putting in the work; he rarely showing up.

His response to my lengthy text was, "I'll be home this weekend." I had my doubts.

When the weekend rolled around so did Jeremy, dragging a carry-on size bag. I didn't know what he had taken from the house, if anything. And I didn't ask.

After spending some time in his room, Jeremy came out to the deck and said, "I need to tell you something." I braced myself and told him to go on. "I'm not even supposed to tell you this," he continued, "but there's no other way to explain what's going on."

I literally held my breath. Jeremy dropped his head and told me that in early February, he'd stopped in the parking lot of a closed business with Richelle. The police came to see what was going on. That's when the cops discovered drugs and arrested them both.

"Drugs?" I gasped. "What kind of drugs?"

Jeremy shrugged. "Some pills and a little weed."

Instead of locking them up, the police offered a way they could "help themselves out"—by becoming a CI for the local sheriff's office A CI stands for "confidential informant. It's a person the police solicit to do undercover drug buys from dealers so that they can then arrest the dealer. (I had no idea what Richelle had to do as part of her agreement and I don't care.)

Instead of asking for a lawyer, which Jeremy was educated enough to know, he agreed to become a CI. He claimed that his fear of me finding out about his arrest, the shame and damage it might cause our business plus his anxiety that he wouldn't be able to see his step kids anymore led to his decision. He panicked and said yes to the CI deal.

I know Jeremy was scared to death. The thought of him going to jail was beyond his comprehension. So, Jeremy agreed to be wired and make drug buys for the police. He had to make three successful drug buys to in order to have his charges dismissed. Jeremy had already done two. Now he had to make himself available when the cops called him and wanted him to make the final buy.

When Jeremy told me this, my heart dropped into my stomach. I'm a super fan of crime TV, so I know the drill. I've watched so many of these shows that I'm aware of how dangerous it is for even an undercover cop to go into that situation, much less a guy who has no previous experience. I was shocked that the police would recruit a civilian with no training and no history of any crime and put them in such a volatile situation.

I immediately said, "We're going to see a lawyer!" To my surprise, Jeremy didn't give me any pushback.

•

After researching the criminal attorneys in town, I found the one who had the best reputation and handled the big cases in the area. When I spoke to him, he told me that it could cost up to $15,000 to take on a case like Jeremy's. I couldn't get access to that much money all at once without jeopardizing the business. But I told him that I could come up with half. Next, I called a very good friend and explained what I needed. Within thirty minutes, the money was wired to my account.

The day Jeremy and I met with the lawyer, he permitted me to be in the room. Maybe this was because I was the one with cash in my purse. But whatever the reason, I was grateful.

When the attorney asked Jeremy about his criminal history, he was surprised that my son had no criminal past. As the conversation went on, the attorney asked Jeremy what drugs they'd found and charged him with. Jeremy ticked off a laundry list of drugs. The last one he mentioned was heroin. Jeremy's eyes were downcast; he couldn't even look at me.

Heroin!! My heart sank. I just couldn't imagine Jeremy messing with heroin. Maybe some pain pills occasionally but never heroin.

The lawyer's recommendation was for Jeremy to go ahead and finish up the CI agreement instead of trying to get his drug charges reduced or risk the possibility of going to jail. I was opposed to it because of the danger. I had also lost trust in the police since they had so little regard for my son's safety to put him in a situation like that in the first place.

The attorney assured me that he trusted the police to uphold their end of the deal. Plus, it would be much better to get Jeremy's charges dismissed through the DA instead of by the court. We paid the attorney his $500 an hour rate and went on our way. I was shaken to my very core.

On the way home, I said to Jeremy, "What the hell? You never said word about heroin." As he drove, Jeremy insisted he'd told me about heroin being part of the deal. I was sure he didn't. Was my son gaslighting me?

I firmly explained to Jeremy that had I heard about the heroin, I would have remembered it. I would have been upset on a whole different level.

I was in shock. My whole world was spinning around me. I was angry. I was scared. And I was as sad as I had ever been. I felt like my life, that our lives, were spinning out of control.

Waiting for the police to call Jeremy to finish the CI agreement kept my anxiety level sky high. On top of that, I was also running a business with thirteen employees, who, by the grace of God, were wonderful people who would do most anything for me.

I didn't know how much I'd come to rely on them. But I would very soon.

19

Midnight Confession

About a week after he returned home, Jeremy sat down and told me that he'd fulfilled his agreement with the sheriff's office. He said it happened when he was away for a short time. Jeremy met up with someone who was obviously an addict and a small-time dealer. The fellow told Jeremy that he wanted to rob a mom-and-pop pharmacy in a town nearby. Jeremy agreed to do the robbery with him and they proceeded to iron out the details.

Unbeknownst to the lowlife, Jeremy called the sheriff and told him what was going on. They promptly set up the arrest strategy.

The thug planned to use Jeremy's truck to commit the robbery, use a chain to pull down the pharmacy's doors, then take all the narcotics inside the drug store. It seemed like a fool-proof plan. But just as the two of them were initiating the break in, the police came from all directions and took them into custody.

Jeremy handed me his phone and pulled up the local news article about the "attempted robbery." It seemed like an important arrest as the drugstore had large amounts of narcotics in stock. The authorities believed that if the thieves had succeeded in getting the doors pulled off, most likely the store's entire wall would have come down as well. Right behind it is where their million-dollar pill packaging machine was located. Jeremy's paperwork was now ready to go to the DA so his charges could be dropped.

It took a couple of phone calls and a few days before my son was told that he could go to the courthouse and get the dismissal in writing. To say we were relieved is an understatement. Everything was taken care of. Jeremy's slate was wiped clean and he could start all over again. He planned to get counseling and medication to curb his addiction once and for all. I was as sure as could be that Jeremy had learned his lesson and this dark chapter of his life was over.

•

June turned to July. We had a huge July 4th barbecue planned at our house for all of our employees and their plus-ones. Jeremy always bought tons of fireworks. After we ate, swam and played corn hole and badminton, he set up for his fireworks display. (Maybe I'd given him the bug when I bought him all those fireworks when he and I were on the run from Brooks when Jeremy was little.) Most of the time, Jeremy's show ended up being almost as big as the one put on by a small town. He got totally into it. But that's the way my son did everything—full on, full of passion.

As I was preparing for the party the next day, my phone rang. It was Jeanne, my best friend of sixty-five years calling me from Kansas City. Jeanne told me that her son Peter was dead. Dead at forty-five. I was dumbfounded.

This hit closer to home than I cared to admit. Peter was Jeremy's first playmate and part of the Tribe. I knew Peter had struggled with drugs and alcohol for years. He'd been to multiple rehabs with limited success. But for the last twelve months or so, Peter seemed to be back on the straight and narrow. He'd returned to his job as a firefighter and had recently married.

Tearfully, Jeanne recounted how on July 3, Peter said his I-love-yous and headed out for work. But instead of going to work, he went to a liquor store, checked into a motel and took his own life. I ached for Jeanne, her husband Dominic and the entire family. I was there the day Peter was born, and I promised Jeanne that I would be there the day her son was buried.

Because we had everything prepared for the July 4th barbecue the following day, Jeremy and I decided to go on with it as planned. But our hearts weren't into it. I tried my best to enjoy the day and be a good hostess but my thoughts were with Jeanne and Dominic. I needed to get to her side as soon as possible to be there for her. The next morning, I flew to Kansas City.

•

Jeremy and I made a deal that whenever I called or texted him, he would answer me within fifteen minutes. Every day I was in Kansas City, I texted him in the morning to check in and sometimes called in the evening as well. Not only did this keep us connected but it kept my fears that he was using drugs again at bay.

The morning after Peter's funeral, I texted Jeremy and got no response. I waited about twenty minutes and tried again. I called his phone and it went directly to voice mail. I continued calling and left several frantic messages. I was beginning to get a sinking feeling in my gut that I couldn't ignore.

In an attempt to assure myself that Jeremy hadn't gotten in more trouble, I checked the sheriff office's website for any recent arrests or bookings. I was relieved to find nothing there. I knew Richelle was in jail in another parish two hours away so Jeremy couldn't be with her. But somehow, I just couldn't shake the feeling that whatever was going on was connected to that witch.

Just to be sure, I checked the sheriff's website in the parish where Richelle was jailed. And sure enough, Jeremy had been arrested and booked that morning. To say I was livid is an understatement!

I called Kyle, my business manager and friend, and told him to get $800 out of the bank. He'd then take it to Jeremy's ex Jennifer, who would bail him out and bring him home. I asked Jennifer not to tell Jeremy that I was on my way back from Kansas City.

After that, I called the airlines and booked the next flight to Louisiana. I had to land at an airport an hour and half away but it was the only flight I could get that same day. Kyle said he'd come pick me up at the airport and drive me back home. Of course, my return ticket was now no good so it cost me another $600 to get that one-way flight home but it was worth every penny.

I guess I was in shock because I can't even remember the flight back. I found myself getting off the plane and Kyle hugging me tight. He didn't say a thing and I loved him for that.

I had no idea what Jeremy was even arrested for but it didn't matter; he had put himself right back in a really bad situation. I thought he had cut off all communication with Richelle. She'd gone to jail in June in connection with drug warrants and she had other warrants out on her besides. So, I was relieved thinking Richelle was totally out of the picture. But obviously, that wasn't the case.

When Kyle and I got to the house, Jeremy was outside on the deck. His ex Jennifer was there as well. I practically flew from the car port to the house and then was through the French doors to the deck. When I saw Jeremy sitting there, my anger boiled over. I flew into a rage!

I went over and just started pounding him. I hit him anywhere I could reach. Jeremy hung his head in shame and took my beating like a dog who knew he'd done wrong and deserved the whupping. I kept shouting, "You look at me!" But he couldn't.

How in God's name could Jeremy even *think* about doing something that could get him arrested? I just kept hitting him, crying and yelling until finally, I stopped. I ran to the edge of the deck and vomited over the side. I threw up until I had nothing left inside me. Then all I could do was retch. It was horrible.

•

The next day, when I recovered, Jeremy told me that he'd been arrested for introducing contraband into a jail. It seems he hadn't broken contact with Richelle, even while she was incarcerated. Instead, she'd talked him into putting a Suboxone strip under the stamp on a letter and mailing it to her at the jail. Suboxone a strong medication to treat opioid addiction.

I knew then that Jeremy's mind wasn't working properly. Why? Because he knew darned well that Suboxone, which is used to block opioids, wouldn't get anyone high. Why in the world would he do something like that? There was no rational explanation and Jeremy didn't attempt to provide one.

When the prison discovered the contraband hidden under the postage stamp, the warden called Jeremy and asked him to come in. Innocently my son did, admitted what he had done and was subsequently arrested.

Of course, now Jeremy was going to need another attorney. One who could go before the court in the parish where he was arrested. We managed to find a lawyer to consult with Jeremy but he required a $7,000 retainer. What choice did I have? I shook my head, wrote him a check then left the room. The attorney and Jeremy discussed the case.

Later, Jeremy explained that he had to attend a preliminary hearing and his lawyer would advise him from there. Because Jeremy had no criminal record (remember, his previous offense had been expunged), the lawyer was pretty sure Jeremy could get either a diversion program where he would receive treatment, or at most, probation.

But regardless of his punishment, Jeremy was going to carry an arrest record for the rest of his life. In his moments of rational thinking, I believe this bothered Jeremy more than I knew.

20

Gone

Facing the fate of having a criminal record plus knowing how disappointed and angry I was really affected Jeremy's frame of mind. Because of it, he wasn't spending much time with Will and Emma, and they wanted to know why. Personally, I thought Jeremy was lucky that his ex-wife Jennifer didn't cut him off from them entirely but I think my son was too down to realize it. Jeremy was also looking at the distinct possibility of having to file for personal bankruptcy. I think it all became too much for him. I was reaching my breaking point too.

•

On July 18, Jeremy was supposed to go to the Escape Room and help with some routine maintenance. He was scheduled to meet an employee there at two that afternoon. At about two-thirty, the employee phoned me and said that Jeremy hadn't showed up. I thought this was odd because Jeremy had been on his best behavior since his arrest.

When I couldn't reach Jeremy by phone or text, I opened my phone app to get a "real time" location on Jeremy's phone. It showed that he was just up the road from the Escape Room. Could he possibly be asleep in his truck? Or something worse?

I asked our employee to drive up the street to check if he saw Jeremy's truck anywhere. When he said he didn't see it, I started getting anxious. Jeremy had probably turned off his phone. Damn. I don't think he had ever turned off his phone before. Jeremy had it with him 24/7.

My brain immediately skipped to all the negative things this could signify. In an attempt to figure out where Jeremy might be, I tried to retrace his steps. I started off looking for a money trail. You know, checking various banks and business accounts, even though he didn't have direct access to them. I looked at the company account even though I knew he couldn't get his hands on the debit card or checks.

But low and behold, when I pulled up the business account online, it showed that Jeremy had gone to the bank a few hours earlier and had written a counter check there. He was a co-owner on those accounts, so of course he could write a check! The odd thing was, Jeremy only cashed a check for $300. I suspected he was going on a drug binge and thought that maybe he took such a small amount of money so he could limit his use—and my level of anger.

I had to get to the bottom of this. I kept calling people and places, trying to find where Jeremy could be. In one way, this was like an Escape Room puzzle. The only difference was that I had no clue where this was going to lead—and maybe I didn't want to find out. But when I did find out the reason for Jeremy's disappearing act, I knew it wouldn't be good.

Next, I called Kyle, my faithful business manager, and asked him to call a locksmith. I wanted Kyle to have the Escape Room locks changed immediately then come pick me up so Kyle could take me to the bank. If Jeremy wasn't thinking clearly—and obviously, he wasn't—I knew I had to protect the business. I couldn't allow him access to the building or to the bank accounts. I had no idea he might do. I couldn't let him wreck what we'd worked so hard creating.

The realization that I hadn't a clue what Jeremy was thinking or what he was possible of doing was absolutely gut wrenching. He and I had always shared total trust and had been in tune with each other before Jeremy's alternate life, his drug-addled life, started. This was a whole different animal. And I didn't know what this animal was capable of.

•

Kyle and I went to the bank, shut down the accounts and had the locks changed. I also took Jeremy off the State registration as an owner of the Escape Room. It sounds drastic, I know, but as the old saying goes: fool me once, shame on you; fool me twice, shame on me. I lived by that credo. Besides, I had thirteen other people depending on me, expecting a paycheck. Had Jeremy decided to take more money out of the bank, he could have emptied the accounts and our employees would have been screwed.

When I spoke to Jeremy's ex Jennifer, I asked if Emma and Will had heard from him. Jennifer said they had. At a little before 2 p.m. Jeremy sent a text to both kids. Three simple words: "I love you." It must have been just before my son turned off his phone. That immediately took my fears from drug binge to suicide.

My mind skipped to Jeanne and Dominic's son Peter, and how he had taken his life because he was powerless against his addiction. I prayed this hadn't happened to my Jeremy. But it would be just like Jeremy to leave his step kids with an "I love you" message as his last communication with them. Because of what Jeremy had been going through, there was a good chance he was suicidal.

All that day and into the night, I tried to find Jeremy. Friends drove around to every part of town he could possibly be, visiting all the places he might go. I was on the phone non-stop, using Jeremy's call record log, reaching out to any and all of his contacts listed there.

It was very late at night when I realized that there was no one left to call, no place left to search. I felt so hopeless. All I could do at this point was lay in my bed and wait for a knock at the door. Mentally wrecked and physically exhausted, I dreaded the police showing up to tell me Jeremy was dead.

After a fitful night, I woke up and rushed to Jeremy's room, hoping to find him fast asleep in bed. But no such luck. It wasn't a bad dream after all. Then I checked the carport to see if his truck was parked there. Maybe, just maybe, he was crashed out in his truck. But the carport was empty. Jeremy hadn't come home.

I grabbed my phone and started over again. I had everyone, including the police, looking for Jeremy. I pleaded silently, "Please, God, let him be alive." I just couldn't bear the thought of my son being found dead somewhere from an overdose. How could I go on living?

In my head, I rehashed every conversation Jeremy and I'd had in the last few months as I waited and waited. Each passing hour made me more and more frightened that Jeremy might not ever be coming home. I spent the day on the phone, checking to see if maybe he had turned his phone on at any time. Then I started praying.

•

Day turned to night. Jeremy had been gone nearly thirty hours. I know that doesn't sound like a long time for an adult to be missing but when they're a drug user, every minute of those hours is like a day. Your very being just gets heavier and heavier with dread.

I sat on the deck and stared at the dark sky. And prayed. And prayed some more.

I called Jennifer one more time, hoping that maybe Jeremy had texted Will and Emma again but he hadn't. Jennifer and I were in the midst of discussing any possible places or people we might have overlooked. As we were talking, I looked up to see a figure coming from the carport toward the deck. Jeremy was home!

I hollered to Jennifer, "He's home!" I put down my phone then ran toward Jeremy. We nearly collapsed in each other's arms. I cried and hugged him, telling him how scared I was and how much I loved him. Jeremy almost toppled over like a tree, his big frame towering over me. He felt good in my arms. I thanked God for answering my prayers.

As Jeremy and I made our way to the deck, I noticed that he had two business size envelopes in his hand. I wasn't concerned about what they were at that time—I had so much else on my mind—but as I think back on it, I'm pretty sure they were suicide letters to me and the kids. The envelopes disappeared shortly afterwards so I never learned what was inside them. And I never will.

When I think back about that day, I wish I had read those letters. Maybe they would have helped me understand what brought this bright, successful, kind man to this point in his life. But the contents of the envelopes were never offered to me, so I never knew. I'm still trying to understand Jeremy's descent into addiction. Why it happened and how. I still can't.

•

That afternoon, my son and I spent some time on the deck, just talking. Jeremy was never religious. Although he was baptized as a baby, he was never active in any church. But he sure talked to God when he was gone those thirty-some-odd hours.

With some difficulty, Jeremy described where he was and what had gone on during the time he was AWOL. He said that he parked in an out of the way place so he could start using the heroin he'd bought with the $300 he'd withdrawn from the bank. Besides the heroin, Jeremy took twenty-six anti-depressants that had just been subscribed for him. And he waited.

A drug cocktail like that could kill a horse. Looking back, Jeremy said he believed that there were only two reasons he survived. One was that he kept nodding off then waking up to vomit. That went on until the drugs were out of his system. It was like having your stomach pumped, I guess.

And the second reason was God.

Jeremy proceeded to relay an unbelievable story. I have no idea whether it was true or a figment of his dope-filled brain. But here it is…

Jeremy said that as he was driving home that night, he saw what he believed to be a church. It was a building with three tall crosses in front of it. Jeremy pulled over and thought to himself, 'Yeah, God, where are you in all of this?'

Jeremy looked at me, his eyes heavy with tears, and said, "Mom, I swear I heard the voice of God answer me. Not like in a dream, but I could actually hear Him speak. And He said, 'No, son, it's not your time.'"

After a few minutes, Jeremy realized that the building wasn't a church at all, but a two-story structure set back from the road. The "crosses" were actually three telephone poles lined up in such a way that they looked like crosses in the dark. God's way of getting my son's attention? I'd like to think so.

By then, Jeremy and I were both exhausted so we agreed to continue our talk in the morning. But first, I explained to Jeremy that there were things he needed to do in order for me to feel like I could go to sleep. He agreed.

I took Jeremy's phone, his money and the keys to his truck. I hid them all in my bedroom, along with my keys and cash. Besides that, I insisted that Jeremy not lock the door to his bedroom. I hugged him tight, kissed him and said, "Don't ever do this to me again. I can't take it." He promised he wouldn't.

Tomorrow, we'd try to figure out what needed to be done. But first, sleep.

I went to bed that night with a prayer of gratitude that my son was still alive and the hope that he could beat this monster that was destroying his brain and his life. And me.

21

Sleepless in Louisiana

Understandably, I slept very little that night. Every possible emotion wracked through my body—but mostly fear. Before daybreak, I got up, fixed myself a cup of tea and went out to the deck to face whatever the day would bring.

Jeremy liked to sleep in so I knew he'd still be in bed. The previous two days must have exhausted him. I decided to let him rest. Maybe it would help him be clearer headed when he woke up.

This early morning alone time also gave me a chance to think about the business. I knew the Escape Room was in good hands with my manager Kyle, but with a staff of young, twenty-somethings, I had to be available to address any need that might arise.

When Jeremy came out to the deck, I knew just by looking at him that he was sick. Dopesick. We didn't do as much talking as I'd hoped. I had so much to say and wanted to hear his side of the story but talking seemed difficult for him.

Jeremy was starting to go through withdrawals. He seemed to be hurting all over, deep down inside. He apologized repeatedly. Knowing how vocal I am, I bet he was also dreading me unloading on him. But I couldn't, not right then, though he probably deserved it.

Instead, I said to Jeremy, "I know you're sick. I can tell by looking at you. So, all I want to say right now is that you have two choices: either you go to rehab or you go nowhere without me and I go nowhere without you. If you're not in rehab, you won't be out of my sight until I feel you can be trusted and that's something that won't happen overnight."

He nodded, listening intently. I kept on, "You change your cell phone number today and you cut off all contact with the people in your drug life. Understood?"

Jeremy simply kept nodding his head. He knew that I would fight for him when he didn't have the strength to fight for himself. He knew I'd always have his back, no matter what. I hope it was a comfort to him.

•

Very quietly, Jeremy went back to his room. That's basically where he stayed for the whole week. He was horribly sick; chills, shaking, stomachache, headache. Heroin withdrawal is not a pretty sight. It was painful for me to see him like that. He barely ate and spoke to no one.

I explained to the kids that Dad had a problem with drugs and was getting them out of his system. Right now, he was too ill to talk to them but as soon as he was able, he would. I could tell by their voices that they were surprised, disappointed and scared. But I assured them that their father loved them very much. Hearing this seemed to make them feel a little better.

I had never seen Jeremy this sick in his life. Even I was feeling sorry for him, despite the hurt and worry he caused, despite the lying and stealing, despite how he almost destroyed our business with his addiction.

At one point, I asked if Jeremy wanted me to take him to the hospital to get help with the detox. He shook his head, "No, I did this *to* myself, so I have to do this *by* myself." I respected him for that.

When Jeremy finally felt well again, we started having daily talks. First, about him going to rehab. He agreed to go but when I called about local facilities, they wouldn't take him on as an inpatient because he was already detoxed. They would only do outpatient therapy.

Because Jeremy already had a relationship with a counselor, we decided that maybe it was best for him to just continue seeing her. I repeated the ground rules I'd laid out when he first came home and Jeremy confirmed that's the way it needed to be.

"I know you're a grown man," I began. "And later, we'll have to discuss boundaries. But until I feel like I can trust you even a little bit, you have to be willing to be totally transparent with me. Including not being on your own at all."

Jeremy replied, "Mom, you have every right to lay down rules that make you comfortable. I messed up and right now, I don't deserve your trust." I had such admiration for the fact that Jeremy admitted to his guilt, to his screwup. A lot of people wouldn't. A lot of people would make excuses and try to place the blame elsewhere. But not my Jeremy. It made me love him all the more.

•

For the next three months, Jeremy and I were back in sync. We discussed everything that had gone on. I asked how he could possibly do something so stupid as to put a needle in his arm, much less touch heroin. He expressed his own disbelief and surprise at what he had done but he tried to explain it to me the best he could.

Like so many people do, Jeremy's addiction started with pills. I'm sure he was supplying Richelle with them too. When his pill habit got too expensive, he started buying heroin, which was cheaper and easier to get.

I told Jeremy how lucky he was that he hadn't gotten into fentanyl, a synthetic opioid that was a hundred times stronger than morphine. It was so prevalent in the area and very dangerous. Jeremy agreed.

He also admitted that if he had gotten away from Richelle like I'd begged him to, he probably wouldn't have ended up where he was. Once again, Jeremy said, "You were right, Mom."

It takes a strong person to admit they were wrong. Jeremy was showing me a depth of character

I never knew he had. I was proud of my son, despite it all.

Jeremy and I talked about the core of his being—his essence, his foundation. I wanted to make sure he knew that I always supported him and that I would never tell him anything that wasn't to his benefit. I think he realized this when he wasn't under the influence but all rational thought leaves once that poison hits your bloodstream.

I struggled to understand Jeremy's addiction. I wanted to know what doing heroin was like, so I asked him. Jeremy shook his head in response. "Mom, you can't imagine what heroin does to you," he sighed. "Once the drug hits, you simply don't care about anyone or anything. In seconds, your troubles, your common sense, your boundaries, your intelligence, all go away. It's pure euphoria. All you want to do is be high! And stay high!"

Trying to grasp what I'd just heard, I asked, "Wasn't it exhausting, living a double life?"

Jeremy replied, "Very."

Somehow, he had managed to be an extremely high-functioning addict. And for some time. I never suspected that Jeremy was on drugs. The people at work never saw him stoned. None of his closest friends knew. Although later, a couple of them said that when they spoke with Jeremy, they noticed a slight difference in him. But they just chalked it up to him being a bit depressed or preoccupied with something.

Of course, I knew something was slightly off with Jeremy but I attributed it to the bad company he was keeping; (i.e., Richelle.) But not once did I link it to heroin, even though I was fairly educated about drugs and drug abuse.

Even now, years later, questions pop up in my mind. What did I miss? How could I not have known?

•

Every day, I made sure to tell Jeremy, if you have the slightest inkling, whim, thought or desire to use, just come to me and say, 'Mom, I'm having a hard time right now,' and we'll do whatever it takes to get you through that moment. Jeremy said he would.

Every night, I made sure that when I went to bed, I kissed him goodnight and hugged him tight. Knowing I almost lost Jeremy, I took advantage of every chance I had to tell him how much I loved him and how proud I was of him.

And I thanked God every night for protecting my son.

22

One Day at a Time

Our day-to-day life changed. I tried very hard to remember that Jeremy was a grown man and not that little boy I still had in my heart. But I still couldn't treat him like the man he had always been due to all of the bad decisions he'd made. This broke my trust in him.

Jeremy and I spent hours and hours talking. We went back through his life and our experiences together, the good and the bad. I apologized for "beating" on him. His response was, "Don't apologize, I deserved it."

He even supported the way I was forced to treat him, adding, "As a matter of fact, you deserve to question everything." Jeremy was so regretful about everything he'd done, telling me, "I'm so sorry I put you through all of this."

When he and I were driving home one night, I stopped and said, "You know, you not only are getting your life back but you're giving me mine back too." It was so wonderful to have normal, intelligent conversation with my son again.

Jeremy and I were trying to look ahead to the future. Of course, I was on high alert all the time, watching for any signs of depression or out of the ordinary behavior. I routinely searched Jeremy's living quarters for anything that shouldn't be there. We both agreed that he needed to be in a different environment, to leave behind the friendships and associations that could lead him back to self-destruction. But could he actually accomplish this?

•

Back in 2013, I started taking yearly vacations to Palm Springs, California to visit my long-time friend Elise. I loved it there and could see myself retiring there. Of course, when Jeremy started the business, things were chaotic, so I didn't talk as much about my retirement dream But I brought it up now, in 2018, when Jeremy was in recovery.

Palm Springs was ripe with opportunity. I mentioned to Jeremy how Elise had said that if Jeremy and I ever moved there, he'd have no trouble starting his own "handyman" business and building a crew into a company. There was a shortage of good, reputable handyman services out in the California desert and people were willing to pay, and pay well, to have work done.

I was totally in love with the city and the weather. The thought of having a friend already there made the idea of moving there even more enticing. Jeremy thought Palm Springs would be a good choice for him, not only as a work opportunity, but it was much closer to the places he panned for gold. The California mountains were also ripe with outdoor recreation spots. Jeremy had some family on his dad's side nearby as well.

Excited, Jeremy and I started formulating a plan to sell the Escape Room in late 2019, take the proceeds and move to California. We'd have enough money to be comfortable until Jeremy could get the handyman business going and settle into a new kind of life.

He and I were so stoked about the idea of starting over again in the desert that we talked about it daily. I wanted it to be something Jeremy could look forward to—and it was. A second chance. A new lease on life.

•

Jeremy and I were constantly focused on rebuilding our relationship. We discussed speaking with a counselor about how we could best establish new healthy boundaries and how to work on regaining trust. We tried to focus on the future instead of the past.

I loved the tradition we started, going out for Mexican food at a local restaurant every Thursday night. I called it "mom and son night dinner." It was a good way for us to get out of the house and enjoy food we both loved. And enjoy each other's company. Taco Thursdays were always just for Jeremy and me. No one else was included. I have such wonderful memories of those nights.

But besides our weekly Mexican restaurant adventure, he and I spent most nights—and days—at home. When the local casino sent a flyer about a Jefferson Starship concert they were hosting, I thought a little musical diversion was in order.

After all, Jeremy and I had a "history" with the band. Originally, Starship was known as Jefferson Airplane. When I was pregnant with Jeremy in 1974, I was first in line to get tickets to their Kansas City concert. More than forty years later, I stilled loved the band.

When I asked Jeremy if he wanted to go to the Starship concert, he thought it sounded like a lot of fun. I guess he'd heard them so much growing up—and in utero—that he appreciated their music. So, I bought tickets for Jefferson Starship's October 12 concert. I was looking forward to spending a Friday night out with my son.

Although I never thought it was possible, I was happy once again. But little did I know, it would be short-lived.

•

Weeks went by. I was continually going through Jeremy's room and keeping very close tabs on him. Slowly but surely, I was beginning to notice that Jeremy was getting back on his feet. In the six weeks since the tight restrictions were put in place, Jeremy spent hours and hours riding the lawn mower all over our three-acre plot, listening to music on his headphones. I suppose it gave him a kind of solitude but he did it so much, he was beginning to mow the dirt!

I knew Jeremy needed to do something productive with his time but I didn't want it spent doing Escape Room stuff. The construction and creative side of the business were the parts he liked. He wasn't interested in the day-to-day mechanics of running an establishment. But was he ready to take on a job? Could I trust him? I guess time would tell. He couldn't keep mowing the lawn forever.

Jeremy knew so many people in the construction industry and had such a good reputation that with one phone call, he was offered a position as a construction manager locally. He and I discussed the parameters of what that would look like. He thought he was ready, and reluctantly, I had to agree that he needed to give it a shot.

After establishing some ground rules, Jeremy went to work in the beginning of September 2018. I thought he was doing well. Will and Emma began coming over again and having sleepovers some weekends. Jeremy's mood was upbeat and positive. I was still checking in with him daily, asking where his head was at and if he was thinking clearly. Jeremy assured me that he was in a good place.

Every chance I could, I told Jeremy how great he was doing and how proud I was of him. To balance it out, I also mentioned that I couldn't go through another bout of addiction. "Neither can I," he'd say. I'll never be sure if Jeremy was using at the time. But to the best of my knowledge, I don't think he was.

Jeremy's new job was going well. He was enthusiastic about the opportunity his friend had given him and seemed to be thriving in his work environment.

On the legal front, Jeremy was still dealing with the criminal charges for sending contraband into a prison but his attorney was fairly certain he could work out a diversion program where the charges would eventually be expunged from his record. So, it looked like Jeremy wasn't going to have to serve any jail time. He knew he'd have to fulfill some punitive terms of the agreement (like community service) but it wasn't anything he couldn't handle.

The fall of 2018, I was back to being Mom and I relished the role. Cooking meals, tending to the home and running the business, mostly be telephone. It was a peaceful, fulfilling existence.

I am forever grateful to Kyle, Katie and all the young people who worked hard at the Escape Room. They were so loyal to the business and to me. Without them, I'm not sure what would have happened to the Escape Room because I was so focused on helping my son get clean and sober. I was feeling more confident that Jeremy was on the road to a successful recovery. But little did I know what the immediate future held.

23

Come October

Come October, things seemed more normal than they had been for years. I still controlled the money and Jeremy agreed to a curfew. I was beginning to see sunlight again.

On October 12, the evening of the Jefferson Starship concert, Jeremy and I decided to have a nice dinner at the restaurant in the casino where the concert was being held. We had a great conversation alongside the meal and the Starship concert was wonderful.

Of course, I knew every word to every song and was out of my seat dancing the whole time. Instead of being embarrassed by his old hippie mom's antics, Jeremy took videos of me dancing. I still have them on my phone.

After the Starship concert, Jeremy and I went over to the merchandise table where the band was sitting. David Frieberg, the only remaining member of the original band Jefferson Airplane, was there. I said to him, "The last time I saw you in concert, I was pregnant with my son here. He's forty-three years old now." David laughed and seemed to appreciate this.

When he and Jeremy shook hands, my son admitted, "I guess you could say I've been a fan my whole life." It was a memorable moment.

As Jeremy and I walked through the casino to leave, I handed him some money. We both played slot machines right next to each other. As the slots do, we won a little then lost a little. We must have played on our initial cash for about an hour, laughing and bemoaning the spin of the wheels.

On the ride home, Jeremy and I talked some more about the logistics of our relocation to California at the end of the following year. We discussed how he would load his truck and trailer with his extensive rock-hounding collection, work tools and equipment. We planned how he would drive out there and possibly store his truck and loaded trailer at his uncle's home less than 60 miles away from Palm Springs in Riverside. Jeremy would find an apartment or condo for us and then fly back to Louisiana where we would both prepare to sell the business, pack up the house and finally make the move. It was a great plan!

•

The next day was Saturday. Repair work was needed at the Escape Room, so Jeremy spent most of the day there. He called me at seven that night and said he was on his way home. I mentioned that

Jennifer had phoned. She wanted to know if Jeremy was still going to pick up his eleven-year-old step daughter Emma to spend the night. He agreed to make the forty-five-minute drive to go get Emma. Then he'd come straight home.

On the way back, Jeremy called and said they were going to stop at Hardy's to get some food. Did I want anything? I told him a burger would be great. About twenty minutes later, Jeremy and Emma arrived at the house.

Ever since she was little, Emma was daddy's girl. She always got her way by sweet-talking Jeremy and he fell under her spell. Without fail, during sleepovers, Emma convinced her dad to let her watch a movie with him in "the big bed." Nine times out of ten, she fell asleep before the movie ended, which ensured that she got to stay in his room.

Around 10:30 that night, I went into Jeremy's room to wish him and Emma good night. I kissed and hugged them both and said, "See ya in the morning light." Then I went to my room and watched TV until I conked out. It was like any other time my step granddaughter slept over.

•

The next morning, I was sitting on the deck enjoying, the fresh, cool air when Emma came out to join me. She sat down and we talked. Emma said that she'd been chatting with some people on the internet who she didn't know. I told her how dangerous this was—she had no idea who was on the other end of the chat, no matter how nice they seemed. Emma admitted that it was a pretty dumb thing to do and said that her dad had told her the same thing.

I was glad Emma felt close enough to share just about anything with me. She confided in me that because she and her mom weren't getting along very well, Emma tried her best to ignore the difficult situation around her. The internet was a good way to escape, Emma said. I suggested that she find other things to entertain her, like hobbies or art.

It just so happened that I'd purchased some therapeutic paint-by-number kits that Jeremy and I were planning to do together. I told Emma I'd be happy to show her what we had. She could pick a couple to take home and try out. She agreed that it was a cool idea.

I suppose Emma and I had been talking for about thirty minutes when we went to Jeremy's room to get the paint kits. While we were there, she mentioned, "Dad has been in the bathroom a long time."

I kind of laughed and said, "Well, you know how your dad is. He always stays a long time in the bathroom when he gets up."

Emma agreed. "Yeah, but he's been in there a *really* long time." She went on to say that she heard him get up around 6:30 a.m. then went back to sleep. It was now about nine and her father was still in there. My heart turned to ice.

I started calling Jeremy's name. No answer. I thought, *Okay, maybe he fell asleep on the toilet. He doesn't normally get up that early.*

I looked at the bathroom door. It was slightly ajar. But this wasn't unusual. Since the door was faulty, it wouldn't shut all the way, so it didn't lock.

Emma was standing close by. I asked her to push the door open a little to see if he was asleep. Emma moved the door slightly and immediately started calling for me.

I ran to the bathroom and there was Jeremy, lying on the floor, flat on his back, his arms spread and a needle on the ground beside him. All I remember is screaming and screaming his name. I told Emma to call 911, go to the living room and wait for them there. I didn't want her to see what I was seeing.

When I saw my son lying on the bathroom floor like that, I knew Jeremy was gone. His lips and his fingertips were blue. His eyes were shut. Even though I knew in my soul that he was dead, I couldn't give up. I still had to fight for him.

I got down on the bathroom floor and began doing CPR on my son. I wasn't going to quit, not now. Finally, I got to the point where I was out of breath. I hollered for Emma to get a bottle of water from the refrigerator and bring it to me. Although I didn't want her in there, I knew I couldn't keep going without a drink of water. But I was NOT going to stop.

Maybe when the paramedics arrived, they could give Jeremy Narcan and revive him. Maybe there was still hope.

When Emma brought the water, I told her, "Just pour it in my mouth." She did. Again, I sent her away. It seemed like the ambulance was taking forever. We were less than a mile from their headquarters. What the hell was taking them so long?

A few minutes later, first responders filled the bathroom. One of them took me outside. Emma had already called her mom and shortly after, Jennifer and Will arrived. I'll never forget my big, six foot tall, 230 pound, fourteen-year-old grandson grabbing me and crying like a baby.

Next thing I knew, a policeman came outside and quietly said, "Ma'am, I think you know he's gone." I nodded my head. I couldn't speak.

•

In my heart, I know that Jeremy didn't intend to die that day.

There's a saying in the recovery community: "He wanted to get high; he didn't want to get dead." And I think that's exactly what happened with my son.

At the edge of the tub were his cigarettes, lighter, ashtray and an unopened bottle of orange soda. I fully believe that Jeremy intended to get a buzz, have a smoke, sip on some soda then continue with his day. I don't know for certain if this was the first time Jeremy had used since getting clean. But I believe his infected brain convinced him that he could do "a little bit" and stay holed up in the bathroom until his high wore off.

What Jeremy didn't know is that the heroin he bought was laced with fentanyl. It was a fatal cocktail. The police said he died instantly.

•

I have jagged fragments of memories about that day. For instance, I recall that at some point, people started arriving at the house. But I don't know exactly who came or when they got there. However, I do remember making two phone calls. One to my sister Berta in Montana, who was Jeremy's godmother as well as his aunt. The other was to my best friends Jeanne and Dominic in Kansas City, remaining members of the Tribe who had lost their son Peter to suicide three months earlier. I know I made other calls but most everything else was hazy.

It took several hours for the coroner to come. I didn't go back into the house during that time. I now regret that I didn't go inside to kiss Jeremy goodbye. But I knew I couldn't handle it.

I never saw my beautiful son again.

•

October 14, the date of Jeremy's death, happened to be his dad David's birthday. Now they were together again. But October 14, 2018 is also the day my world came crashing down, shattering into pieces.

I wanted the earth to open and swallow me up. I didn't want to live without my son. Through the years, I'd sworn that if anything happened to Jeremy, they may as well dig the hole a little deeper and put me in there with him. I started praying fervently that I would die.

Most of the following week was a blur. My friends from Kansas City arrived. My best friend from Kansas came too. My sister Berta in Montana and my niece Shellie from Kansas were there as well. Shellie and I always had a very warm relationship and she was Jeremy's closest cousin.

Somehow, my friends and family managed to get me through the week. But how would I get through the rest of my life?

•

Five days after his death, on Friday October 19, we held a service for Jeremy. So many people came and spoke about him. All the employees from the Escape Room walked in together with their significant others. My workers proudly wore the T-shirts that were their uniform. I was totally surprised when several of them got up and spoke so kindly of my son.

Linda, Jeremy's best female friend, came from North Carolina with her daughter. Linda was devastated. Letters were read from Jeremy's good friends who couldn't be there. The memorial was a very touching tribute to him.

I brought home Jeremy's ashes in a beautiful wooden box. It lives on a shelf in my bedroom. That and my memories are all I have left of my baby boy Jeremy.

My world changed forever the day Jeremy overdosed. I lost my only child, my best friend, my roommate and my business partner in an instant. And today, more than four years later, my mind still has trouble accepting the unacceptable.

People talk about "moving on," "closure" and "finding a purpose." I don't believe I will ever be able to do any of those things. I wake up each morning and wonder when it will be over.

But other days, I think that maybe I *do* have a purpose. Maybe my purpose is to tell Jeremy's story. Maybe it will be a comfort to other grieving parents who have lost their children to addiction. Maybe hearing Jeremy's story will show them that they're not alone. That a lot of us are out there. And that it's not their fault.

If I can save just one child from addiction, if I can help just one parent recognize the signs, if I could save just one life, then that is my purpose.

Epilogue

The Sunday evening after Jeremy's service, everyone from out of town left Louisiana and went back to their own lives. Everyone except me. My life as I knew it had ended.

When it was all over, it was only Shellie and me. I had already decided that I was going to leave Louisiana as Jeremy and I had planned. But now I was moving to Palm Springs alone. After a big loss like the death of a child, people say, "Don't make any major decisions for a year." But I just couldn't stay in Louisiana. Especially since Jeremy and I had intended to move to out to California at the end of 2019. I was only doing it sooner. And without my son.

The idea of sunshine all year 'round appealed to me. Especially now. Jeremy and I had wanted to start over in the desert. Now I would do it on my own. Well, not totally on my own, because my friend Elise lived in Palm Springs. At least I had someone who cared about me there.

I don't know how I could have gotten through the first six weeks after losing Jeremy without my niece Shellie. She went to work like she was on a mission. Shellie actually *was* on a mission; a mission to keep me alive. A mission to keep me from going to be with Jeremy. I truly didn't want to live anymore.

But instead of letting me focus on dark thoughts, Shellie forced me to roll up my sleeves beside her and concentrate on packing up the house. Together, we sorted out Jeremy's room. I called the kids to come by with their mom to take anything they wanted. The clothes that remained, Shellie and I took to a men's shelter. It was easier to let go of most of Jeremy's possessions because at the same time, we were packing mine.

The biggest hurdle facing Shellie and I was dealing with Jeremy's work equipment and tools. A large shed was filled to capacity with them. It was so packed that you had to remove things to even get inside. There was so much expensive tools and power equipment, a twenty-year collection worth of gear.

Shellie asked her husband Dan what he thought we should do. Dan was familiar with these types of tools because he worked in the railroad industry. He thought Jeremy's equipment was much too valuable to give away or dump. During the next six weeks they helped me clean, check, package and price Jeremy's tools.

We had a huge yard sale. There was so much stuff, Shellie actually organized it into separate "departments." There were so many departments, we hired the Escape Room employees to man them. The equipment sale was very successful.

•

Given my state of mind, Dan was adamant that he and Shellie wouldn't leave my side until they delivered me and my possessions to California and handed me off to Elise.

Again, I was surrounded by angels, people who looked out for me when I didn't have the ability or desire to look out for myself.

Elise was a godsend too. She looked at a place in Palm Springs that I'd found online. Afterwards, she immediately called and said I should take the apartment. It was a very nice two bedroom, two bath setup in a great complex very close to the downtown area. And even better, it was only a few minutes from Elise's house.

I made arrangements for the utilities to be turned on and booked a moving truck. Dan drove the truck and towed Shellie's car. Shellie and I followed in my car. Although it was a long trip, it was drama free. I was very grateful for that. I'd had enough drama to last a lifetime.

We arrived in Palm Springs on November 28, 2018.

I was now based in California but I still had a functioning business in Louisiana. Kyle, my manager, was running the Escape Room onsite. He made major decisions based on our frequent calls. Our employees, who were basically kids, were remarkable. We were a real family who took care of each other. I hit the jackpot when I put this team together.

But I knew that in the long term, I couldn't run a successful business by telephone practically cross country. In January 2019, I got a "what the heck" thought. I decided to reach out to the only other Escape Room owner I was aware of near Lafayette. I knew they were involved in several successful businesses and thought it wouldn't hurt to pitch the idea of them buying my business. To my surprise, they bit and we began negotiating.

Ultimately, I sold the Escape Room lock, stock and barrel for much less than market value. But part of the deal was that they keep my employees for at least ninety days, unless the employee quit. It may have meant less money for me but I walked away with my head held high knowing I did the best I could for my workers. On March 1, 2019, the new owners took control of Jeremy's and my "baby."

•

The only thing that's kept me going the last couple of years was trying to find a way to tell Jeremy's story. I thought that putting it on paper, knowing I had memorialized him in some way would help me heal. And as I grew older and my memories faded, at least I could look back upon this book. At least it would help me remember. Remember Jeremy.

•

Another thing that's kept me going is my grandchildren. My step-grandchildren, really. Although I've never considered them "steps." Jeremy is the only dad they had or ever will have. I'm grateful that Jeremy's ex-wife, their mom Jennifer, has permitted me to be part of Will and Emma's lives. This gives me great joy…well, as close to joy as I can feel.

The kids still live in Louisiana but we talk often. As their GG (which stands for "Grandma Goddess," a play on my old handle, "Poker Goddess," but these days, it's pretty much morphed to "Geeg"), I still try to spoil them long distance. I'm very proud of those two. They're great kids.

As I write this, Will is a senior in high school and Emma is a sophomore. They've both matured so much in the last four years. I try to channel Jeremy when I give them advice. In their minds, I know they always consider "what would dad say?" when trying to make a big decision. I hope they never lose that.

I'm very aware that at my age, I may not be here for much longer. But I believe that the positive influence and lessons Will and Emma have learned from Jeremy and me will serve them well throughout their lives. That is my hope, my prayer. And I have faith that they will never make the same mistakes their dad did.

•

In October 2020, my nephew Dan retired from the railroad. He, Shellie and I decided that for many reasons, they should move to Palm Springs and share my apartment. It turned out to be a beneficial arrangement for all three of us. I am thankful for my niece and nephew's presence in my life. It's very hard to be alone and lonely.

•

My wish and my prayer are that someone will pick up this book and find themselves lost within the pages. That my story, intertwined with Jeremy's story, will touch them in some way. That it will strike a chord with them, ring so true to them that it might, just might, save one family the grief and misery that has become my way of life.

I miss Jeremy every day. Every. Single. Day. When I cook his favorite foods or hear a certain song on the radio, when someone tells a satirical joke I know he would like (or tell himself) …well, I see my son's dimples, his beautiful smile.

Sometimes, just for a moment, I forget that Jeremy is dead and feel like he's in the next room. I have to stop myself from going there to tell him something.

Then, when I remember that my son is gone, I feel a physical pain deep in my chest. It's like a stab, a dagger. I have to struggle to catch my breath and recover. I suppose the truth of the matter is that I don't ever want that feeling, that anguish, to go away. I don't ever want to forget how deeply I cared for my son.

At the end of the day, I'm so glad that the last words I said to Jeremy were "I love you!" Because I did. I still do. I always will.

The contents of this book are Carol Farley's personal memoirs of how she experienced and interpreted the events detailed in this book. They are in no way meant to be a historical accounting. The thoughts, opinions and recollections in no way reflect the opinions of any characters or the publisher.

www.ingramcontent.com/pod-product-compliance
Lightning Source LLC
LaVergne TN
LVHW050643100826
845148LV00011B/1967

* 9 7 9 8 9 8 7 7 9 0 3 7 3 *